WHY? TROUBL

FOOT GAIT & ORTHOTICS

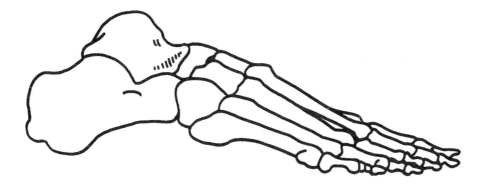

By Dr. Kevin G. Hearon

ACKNOWLEDGEMENTS

My greatest appreciation and grateful thanks to:

My Lord and Savior Jesus Christ who has molded me into a kind, gentle and approachable man over the years. His wisdom is given to those that seek, knock and ask for it.

To my beautiful wife who makes life much more enjoyable and fun.

For the many people that saw the value in what I would share with them and were kind enough to apply it and make a difference in other people.

Teresa Sales at Caxton Printers nurtured the process to completion and cleaned up a number of drawings for greater clarity.

EDITORIAL REVIEWERS

Patrick C. Andersen, D.C., DABCO, CCEP, CCSP
John W. Downes, D.C., CCEP
Marni Capes, D.C., CCEP
Paul Hetrick, D.C., CCEP
Michael R. Krasnov, D.C., CCEP, CCSP
Ronald E. Krugman, D.C., CCEP, CCSP
George Lawrence, D.C., CCEP
Nancy North, D.C., CCEP, CCSP
Keith Rau, D.C., CCEP
Thomas Satterwhite, D.C., CCEP

PREFACE

I wrote this book to help the doctor practically apply this information in the clinic situation from start to finish while giving them options of orthotic production.

Correcting the fixations in the feet to normal glide and position before scanning, casting or molding an orthotic to the normal feet is of great importance.

After all, who would want an orthotic made to their pathological form and position?

TABLE OF CONTENTS

CHAPTER THIRTEEN

CHAPTER FOURTEEN

CHAPTER FIFTEEN

CHAPTER SIXTEEN

CHAPTER SEVENTEEN

CHAPTER EIGHTEEN

CHAPTER NINETEEN

CHAPTER TWENTY

CHAPTER TWENTY ONE

CHAPTER ONE

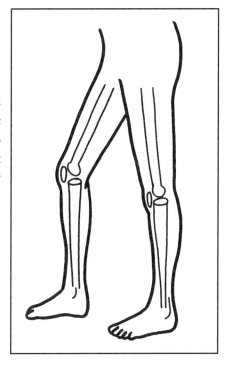

ONCE UPON A TIME

- For centuries man has walked on dirt which absorbed shock and conformed to the shape of the foot and the angle of the foot. This was normal and good to have the earth adapt to man and absorb shock no matter what shape or angle the foot approached the ground at. After all, we are each made very differently with varying angles to our feet.

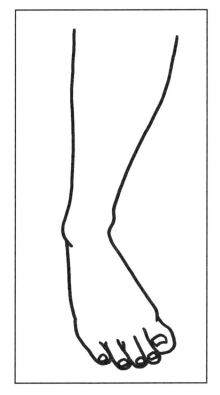

INCREDIBLE SOCIAL EXPERIMENT

- Over the last century or so man has imposed an incredible social experiment on us called, concrete, asphalt and hard wood floors.
- The net result of this experiment is that the ground no longer adapts to us, but we must adapt to the ground. A very hard, flat and unforgiving surface that does not absorb shock well.

SHOCKING RESULTS

- The result of this hostile environment has been increased shock and forced excessive pronation upon over half of the population of the industrialized world. The end result of this excessive twisting of the legs by the feet has lead to large increases in knee arthritis, hip replacements and disc herniation's with no history of trauma.

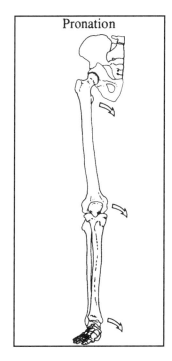

Pronation

DO SHOES FIX THE PROBLEM?

- It used to be that a cobbler really did make shoes specific to a foot and its angle and size. In fact it was 1908 before shoes were made specific to right and left feet.
- That all changed when mass production came of age and could produce shoes much cheaper and faster to shod the masses. Shoes became a generic shape and angle and were no longer person specific.

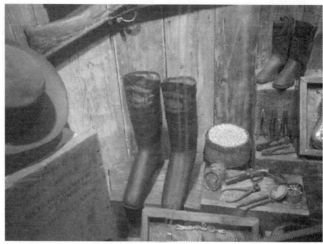

Steamship Arabia sank in 1800s on the Missouri River

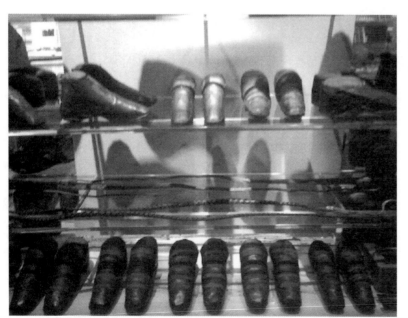

Steamship Arabia sank in 1800s on the Missouri River

THE PROBLEM WITH SHOES

- Vanity for many has trumped functionality and comfort. "If it looks good, wear it" seems to be the theme of some while fads drive the purchasing of many shoes. Most people don't know the difference between a good shoe and a bad shoe. Therefore they are at the mercy of a sales person that frequently acts like they know. But do they?

CHAPTER TWO

WHAT PROFESSION IS BEST SET UP TO HELP?

- There are a number of professions that consider themselves as experts on the feet and how the body adapts if they have had specific foot courses and training.
- I want to focus on one profession which I believe has the best tools to treat most feet before surgery is needed: CHIROPRACTIC. Because chiropractors treat the whole body and can manipulate the bones and soft tissue.

CHIROPRACTIC

- That science and art which utilizes the inherent recuperative powers of the body, and deals with the relationship of the spinal cord and the spinal column and its immediate and distal articulations, and the role of that relationship in the restoration and maintenance of health.
  (Kevin G. Hearon modification of definition)

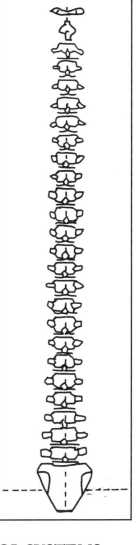

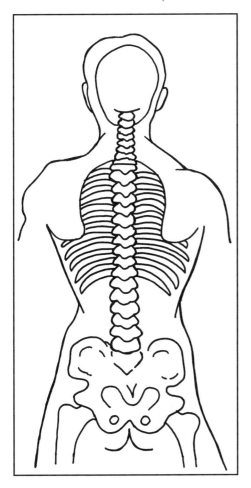

THE TWO MASTER CONTROL SYSTEMS
TOP DOWN & GROUND UP

Chiropractors study the **"NEUROLOGICAL CONTROL SYSTEM"** from the **"TOP DOWN"**, and follow the effects of the brain, spinal cord and its nerve roots out to the organs, muscles and tissues, telling them what to do, when to do it and how much to do it.

We have another system, the **"MECHANICAL CONTROL SYSTEM"** from the **"GROUND UP"**. The feet are much like the foundation of a building that supports the structure above it. Only this structure is a kinetic chain of events controlled by the bones joint angles that are unique to each person.

NEUROLOGICAL CONTROL SYSTEM –
TOP DOWN

Normal neurological function and control from the brain through the spinal canal and nerve roots into the peripheral nerves is dependent upon freedom from impingement, entrapment and inhibition to the adjacent muscular activity. It has both facilatory, excitatory and inhibitive properties.

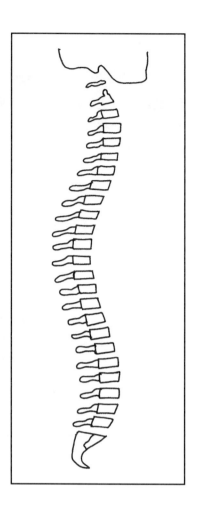

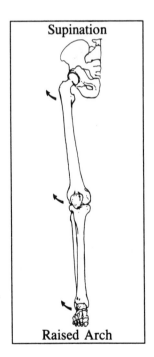

Supination

Raised Arch

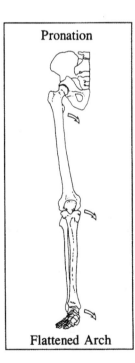

Pronation

Flattened Arch

MECHANICAL CONTROL SYSTEM
GROUND UP

- Kinetic chain events starting with the feet at heel strike goes from supination into pronation and absorbs shock by lowering the tarsal arch and internally rotating the leg, thereby attenuating that shock up the leg into the pelvis and onto lumbar spine.
- Heel raise initiates the supination process from pronation by tightening the plantar fascia and pulling the heel forward thereby raising the tarsal arches and externally rotating the leg when functioning normally.

HARMONY OF SYSTEMS

The neurological function and mechanical function rely on each other for stability.

If either system is out of balance the other will be also.

It is important to have both systems in balance for long term stability, health and patient satisfaction.

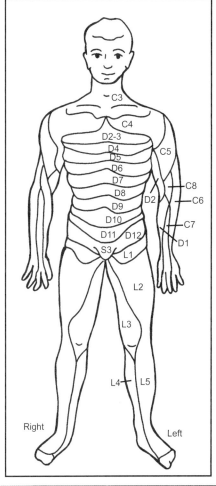

An imbalance could lead to **Fairly Reliable Bob's** Chiropractic Clinic with a disappearing tail light guarantee.

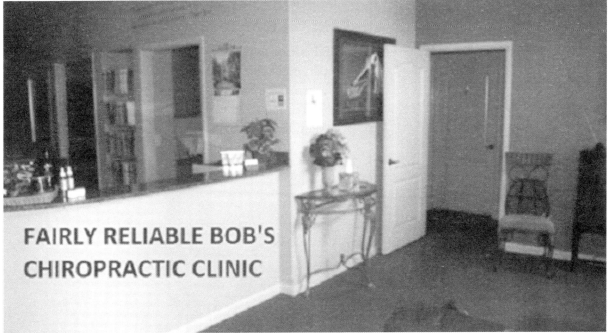

The reputation of "Hit them high – Hit them low, roll them over and take their dough" could result.

CHAPTER THREE

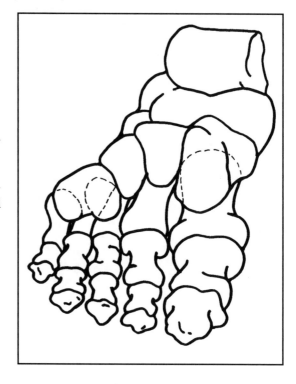

FUNCTIONS OF THE FOOT
(2, P. 6-14; 33, P. 696-757)

- **Adapt to terrain:** Change to the various angles of the surface being contacted.
- **Shock absorption:** Increase length and width. Base for leg and trunk rotation: Pronation and Supination.
- **Stability control:** When is it flexible or rigid?
- Rigid lever for propulsion.

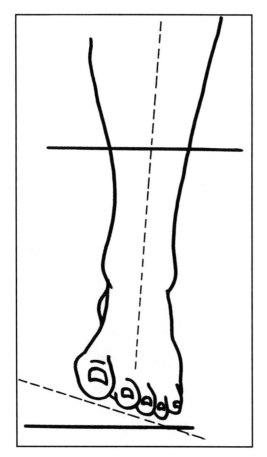

VARIABLE ANGLES OF THE FEET

- The foot in neutral position varies per individual as a perpendicular to the shaft of the tibia.
- Normal is considered from 0 to 4-6 degrees varus. This foot is angled in varus position.
- Many feet are much greater in angulation than normal and must adapt to a hostile flat world.

NEUTRAL POSITION IS NEITHER;

- DORSIFELXION OR PLANTAR FLEXION.
- ADDUCTION OR ABDUCTION.
- INVERSION OR EVERSION.
- IT IS IN BETWEEN ALL OF THESE.
- IT IS NEUTRAL.

The important thing to remember is that neutral is that central point from which ligaments have enough motion to adapt to terrain four to six degrees either medial or lateral.

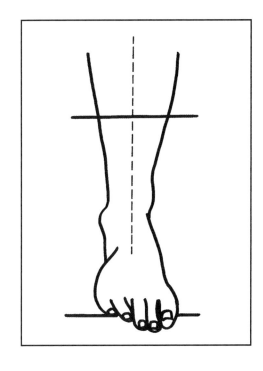

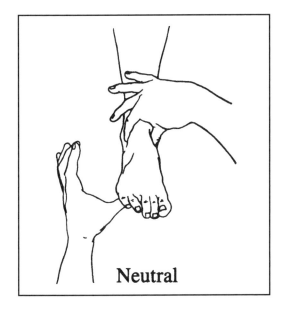

Neutral

NEUTRAL POSITION IS;

- When there is a congruency of the talo-navicular joint.
- Congruency means "being in agreement" and in this case equal indentations on each side of the joint.
- It is the ideal position from which to adapt to terrain.

NEUTRAL POSITION IS;

- Taking a <u>perpendicular</u> to the <u>shaft of the tibia</u> and applying that in relation to the bottom of the foot across the met heads and measuring that angle.
- When in neutral position the terms **VARUS** and **VALGUS** are used to describe the foots position.

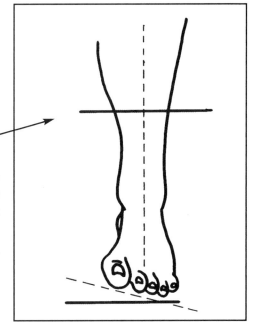

7

CHAPTER FOUR

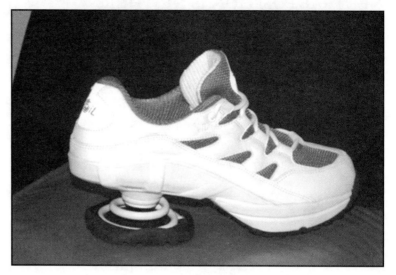

WHAT IS THE PRIMARY SHOCK ABSORBER OF THE BODY?

- Is it NIKE?
- Is it ADIDDAS?
- SAUCONY?
- Z-COIL?
- BERKENSTOCK?

THE PRIMARY SHOCK ABSORBER OF THE BODY IS: FOOT PRONATION

The human foot was designed to rock somewhere between 4 to 6 degrees of inversion or eversion so that it could adapt to terrain. Anything beyond that is either pulling on the ligaments or being adapted by the give of sand or soil. Ligaments can withstand short periods of stress in hostile and hard environments before succumbing to either stretch or tear types of deformation.

Much of the population has foot angles that force the foot to exceed the 4 to 6 degree inversion and eversion of the foot. This usually results in **EXCESSIVE PRONATION** and sometimes excess supination and therefore stretches or tears ligaments.

(43, p.150-153; 46, p. 620-621; 56, p. 576)

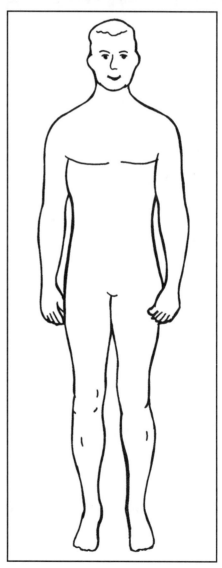

PRIMARY SHOCK ABSORBER ACTION

During normal gait, shock is absorbed almost completely within the foot and the lower extremity. Primarily shock is absorbed by controlled rapid pronation of the foot. The muscle that controls pronation is the posterior tibia. During a normal step shock is attenuated by this muscle slowing the lowering of the medial longitudinal tarsal arch through eccentric contraction. The arch of the foot is therefore lowered gently to the ground instead of slapping the ground. The primary nerve supply to the posterior tibia muscle is the L-5 nerve root.

Could a subluxation of L-5 or an L-4 disc protrusion affect pronation ?

Could a subluxation of the foot affect pronation ?

(43, p.150-153; 46, p. 620-621; 56, p. 576)

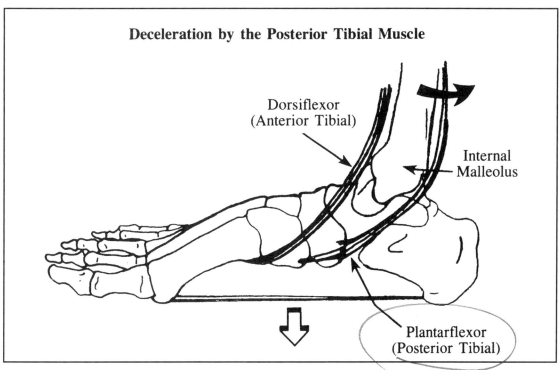

Deceleration by the Posterior Tibial Muscle

Dorsiflexor (Anterior Tibial)

Internal Malleolus

Plantarflexor (Posterior Tibial)

WHAT IS FOOT PRONATION?

- Eversion of the foot?
- Dropping of the medial arch of the foot?
- Abduction of the foot?
- Dorsiflexion of the foot?
- When the heel strikes and the foot flattens out?
- Is it all of the above? Yes.

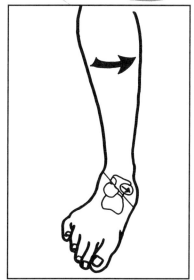

IS FOOT PRONATION NORMAL OR PATHOLOGICAL OR EITHER ONE ?

- Does it increase or decrease shock?
- Can it be excessive?
- Can it be not enough?
- Does it affect anything besides the feet?
- Is it congenital?
- Is it developmental?
- Can it be all of the above? Yes.

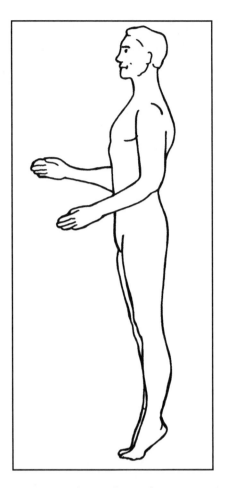

WHAT ARE THE FORCES THAT NEED TO BE ATTENUATED INTO THE FEET EACH TIME I TAKE A STEP DURING PRONATION?

- Walking- One to Three times my body weight. A 200 lb. person creates 200-600 lbs. of force.
- Running- Three to Five times my body weight. A 200 lb. person creates 600-1,000 lbs. of force.
- Jumping- Five to Seven times my body weight. A 200 lb. person creates 1,000-1,400 lbs. of force.

WHAT IS THE PRACTICAL APPLICATION OF NEWTON'S LAWS OF MOTION THAT CONTROL SHOCK ABSORPTION?

- You must increase the surface area of the mass that is striking. Foot length and width.
- You must increase the time it takes to bottom out. (Normal joint glide up and down slowed by the posterior tibia muscle through eccentric contraction while lowering the medial longitudinal tarsal arch.)

HOW COULD SURFACE AREA INCREASE ?

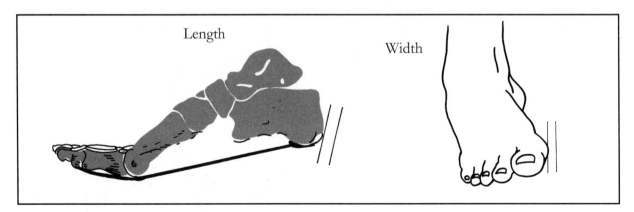

IF JOINTS DIDN'T GLIDE WOULD IT INCREASE SHOCK?

ABNORMAL FOOT FUNC-TION DUE TO EXCESSIVE PRONATION.

- Subluxation of the joints.
- Unstable and fixated arch structure.
- Increased pronatory torques.
- Hypermobile forefoot.
- First ray cannot carry load properly.
- Increased loading of 2,3,4 met heads.
- Increased shearing of met heads.

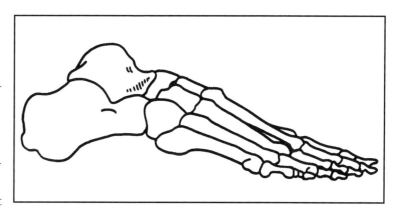

WHICH FOOT IS PRONATED?

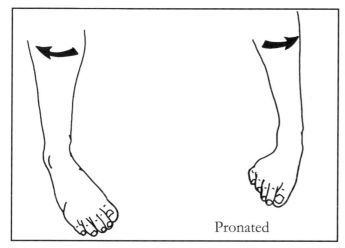

Pronated

ASSUME THE POSITION OF PRONATION & SUPINATION

- Which foot is the pronated foot in your stance?
- In relation to the tibia is the pronated foot dorsi flexed or plantar flexed?

- Is it abducted or adducted?

- Is it everted or inverted?

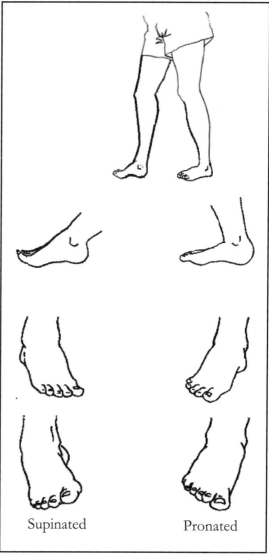

Supinated   Pronated

11

WHAT'S THE REAR FOOT POSITION CALLED?

- Is it plantar flexed or dorsi flexed?

- Is it adducted or abducted?

- Is it inverted or everted?

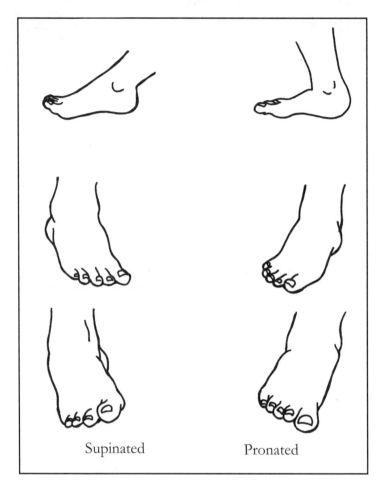

Supinated   Pronated

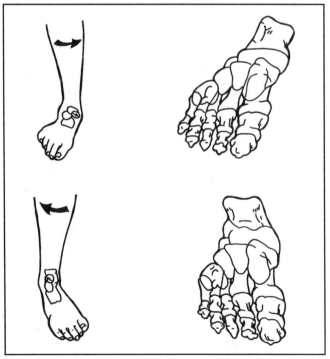

PRONATION AND SUPINATION IS A COMBINATION OF THREE PLANE LINES OF MOTION

- **Pronation:** Dorsiflexion, Abduction and Eversion.
- **Supination:** Plantar flexion, Adduction and Inversion.
(43, p. 159-162)

12

CHAPTER FIVE

SUPINATION

Created by the **Windlass Effect** which is a sailing term that relates to the mechanism of a rope or cable moving heavy objects by winding it around the drum of a *windlass*, which is the metatarsal heads acting as the drum and the fascia acting as the rope. In this case the plantar fascia acts as the rope and lifts the tarsal arch. Since the 1st MTP is much bigger than the other MTP's the medial arch shortens more and raises the medial arch quicker into supination around the windlass.

(8, p 648; 9, p13; 10, p 54,24)

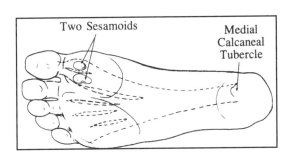

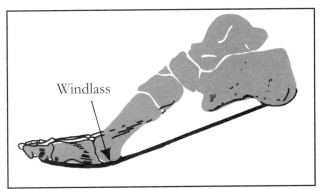

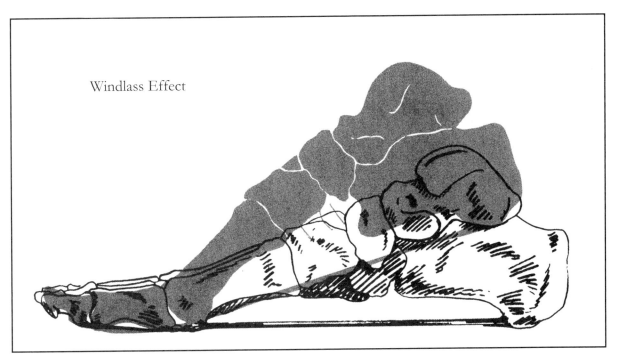

The arch can only raise if the joints can glide and respond to the tightening of the plantar fascia during heel raise.

THE WINDLASS EFFECT: (9,p.13;8,p.648;10,p.54.24)

This mechanism of gait from heel raise to toe off is responsible for supination of the foot and external rotation of the contact leg. It is an involuntary event that normally raises the longitudinal tarsal arch as the foot moves up and over the toes. The flexor hallucis muscle along with the plantar fascia (as it attaches at the plantar surface of the big toe) extends back through the two sesamoid bones, under the first ray and acts as a fulcrum for the plantar fascia. The plantar fascia draws its origin at the medial calcaneal tubercle closer to the toes, thereby raising the medial longitudinal tarsal arch and moving the talar head from horizontal to vertical, externally rotating the tibia and femur.

(41, p 159-160

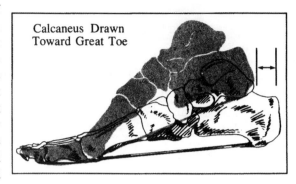

Calcaneus Drawn Toward Great Toe

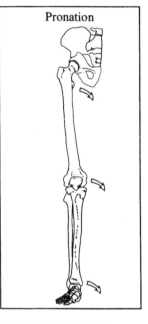

Pronation

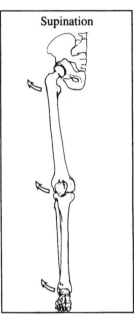

Supination

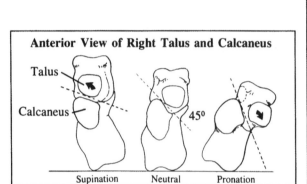

Anterior View of Right Talus and Calcaneus

Talus

Calcaneus

45°

Supination   Neutral   Pronation

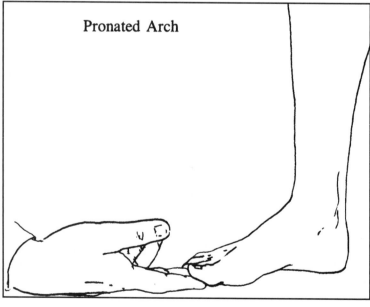

Pronated Arch

To demonstrate the windlass effect, Have a patient stand in front of you with their feet shoulder wide apart and toes straight ahead, grasp the big toe and raise it as high as it will comfortably move. Normal goes up to about 35 degrees when under load. Note what happens to the foot, knee, and leg as you repeat this motion of the big toe. The whole lower limb externally rotates and the arch of the foot raises into supination.

Here you see a normal toe raise and arch raise. The Windlass effect is working well.

Compare this to the other foot function and note any difference. Arches are not always equal in their glide and function and toes do not always raise to the same height.

Limitation of this function is known as *Functional Hallux Limitus.* **It is a limitation of the big toe to dorsiflex while the foot is under load.**

Is this voluntary or involuntary?

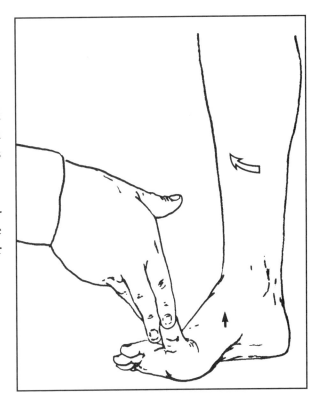

JOINTS MUST GLIDE TO RESTORE THE ARCH AND PREVENT EXCESS TUG ON THE FASCIA

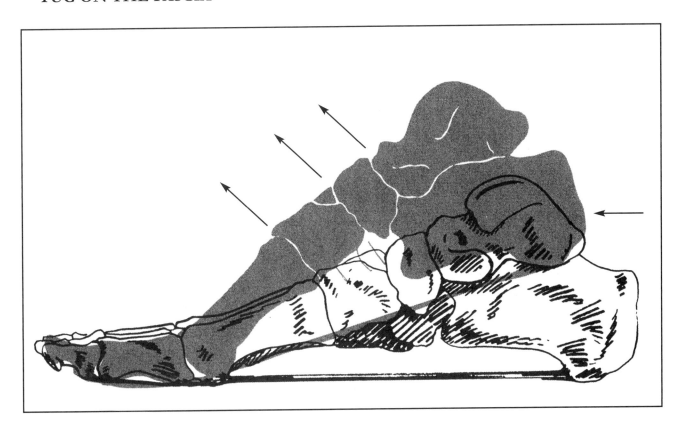

CHAPTER SIX

THE KINETIC CHAIN

Most everything I have shown you has lead up to this point of identifying the series of movements that make up what is known as the **kinetic chain of motion** in the lower extremity. It is important to remember that once muscle fatigue sets in or injury occurs the body will tend to follow gravity and the Ground – Up Master Control System which tends to take over from the Top Down System.

The kinetic chain is simply the sequence of joint coupling that starts at the ground and moves up the leg into the knee, hip, pelvis and spine into the skull. With muscle and structural rehabilitation proper function can usually be restored.

TOP VIEW OF RT. TALUS ON CALCANEUS ARE THE TWO BONES WHICH INITIATE THE KINETIC CHAIN OF MOTION .

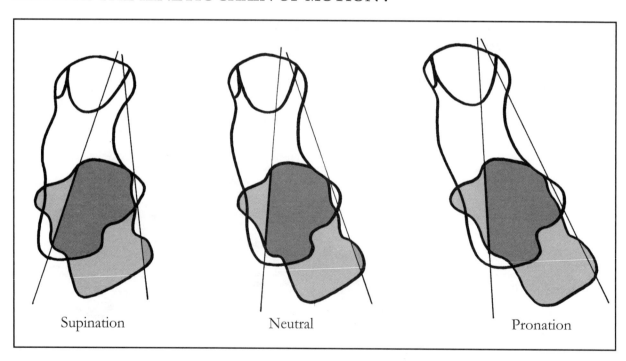

Supination   Neutral   Pronation

ANTERIOR VIEW OF WHOLE FOOT

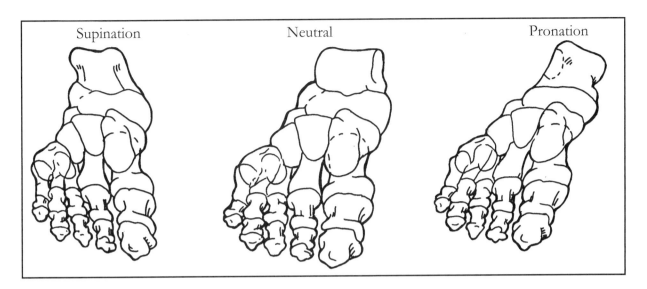

Supination   Neutral   Pronation

BIOTENSEGRITY:

Is the marriage of the network of fascia connective tissue operating with the network of neurons to control the tension level of muscular-articular links.

The fascial net allows the muscles to operate in unison while maintaining a force balance in the body.

(53) M.T. Turvey / Human Movement Science 26 (2007) 657–697

CUBOID CALCANEAL NAVICULAR CUNEIFORM COMPLEX (CCNCC)

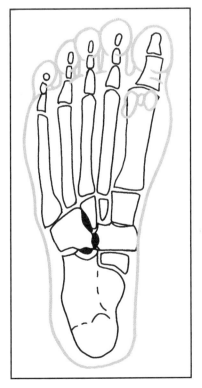

BOTTOM /POSTERIOR VIEW OF RIGHT FOOT

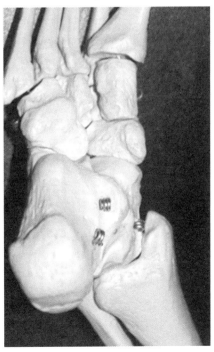

As you observe the gray areas in the middle of the foot you are observing the confluence of facets that control the locking mechanism's of the rear and mid-foot. The cuboid is inferior to all the bones at these junctures and acts as a supporting keystone to these structures.

CUBOID CALCANEAL NAVICULAR CUNEIFORM COMPLEX (CCNCC)

Therefore it is imperative that the CCNCC / LCNC be functional for proper alignment and joint glide to occur. Break down of the ligaments (biotensegrity) and soft tissue on the plantar surface of the foot would compromise the locking points of these bones and result in failure to handle loads properly in the advantaged sequence of motion.

The CCNCC responds to ground reaction forces as the calcaneus begins to plantar flex and the cuboid facet initially engages the calcaneus. As the first ray comes down into the ground, the secondary facets of the navicular and cuneiform engage with the cuboid to create a rigid lever for propulsion.

This is the mechanism that stabilizes the medial column against the lateral column as the foot loads.

(39) kevin.miller@tensegritytech.com e-mail on 6-23-2011

(22) LCNC Lateral Cuneiform Navicular Complex [Glasoe WM, Yack HJ, Saltzman CL. Anatomy and biomechanics of the first ray. Phys Ther. 1999;79:854–859.]

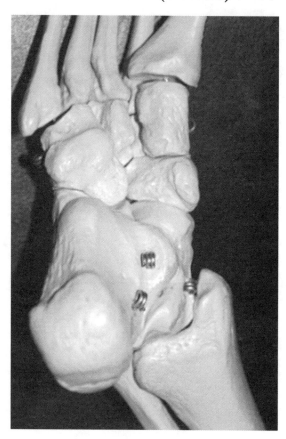

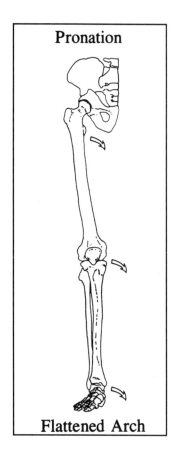

Pronation

Flattened Arch

Pronation is a natural result of the leg and body moving over the foot due to the 45 degree average angle between the talus and the calcaneus. This normally occurs at heel strike as the foot goes from supination to pronation into the mid-stance phase of gait resulting in a flattening of the longitudinal tarsal arch. The talus head moves medially from a vertical position over the head of the calcaneus, to a position horizontal to the head of the calcaneus. The medial twisting of the talus is what internally rotates the tibia and femur above it.

Therefore it is normal for the talus head to fall with gravity down hill from lateral to medial. It is usually an involuntary event that locks the foot.

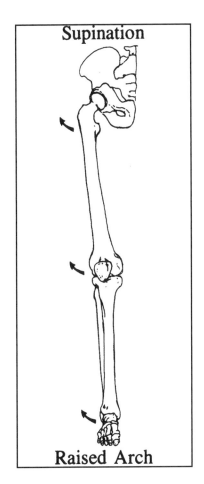

Supination

Raised Arch

SUPINATED

SUPINATION: (43,P.160-162)

This normally occurs during the push-off phase of gait when the foot is fully pronated and the head of the talus is horizontal to the head of the calcaneus. The foot is now in a rigid lever position. Supination begins as the heel raises from the ground. The "Windlass Effect" is activated by the leg and body's forward motion, drawing the rear foot closer to the forefoot and raising the medial tarsal arch. As the arch raises, the talus head raises to the vertical position and externally rotates the tibia and femur.

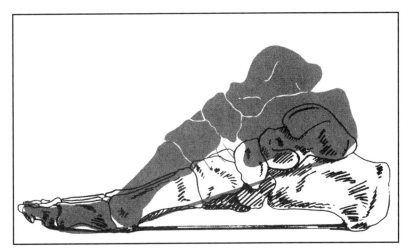

HEEL RAISE

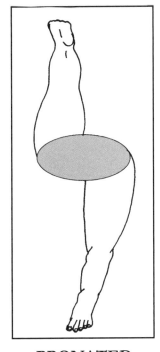

PRONATED

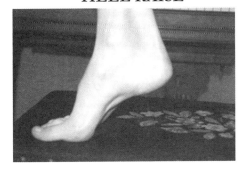

BACK FOOT SUPINATION

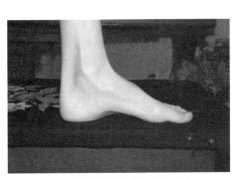

FRONT FOOT PRONATION

HEEL STRIKE

19

TWIST OF PELVIS

Pronation: Rocks the ipsilateral (same side) ilium (pelvis) forward and pulls on the psoas muscle therefore pulling the lumbar spine to the pronated side of the body.

Supination: Rocks the ipsilateral ilium backward and unloads the tug on the psoas muscle therefore releasing the lumbar spine pull.

This tug of war on the lumbar spine due to excess pronation is more than likely the main cause of low back disc protrusions with no history of trauma in my opinion.

(6) (Cambron et al Journal of Manipulative and Physiological Therapeutics Shoe Orthotics for Low Back Pain Month 2011)

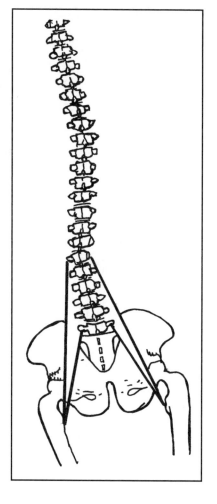

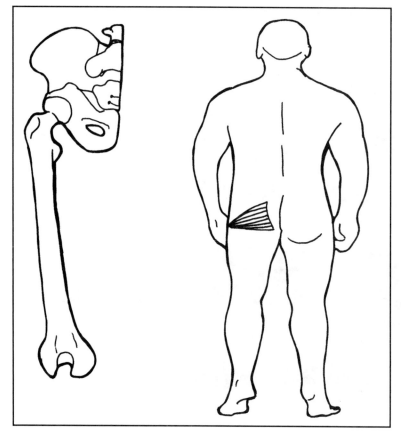

TWIST OF THE HIP

The internal rotation of the left hip can tighten the piriformis muscle which may compress the sciatic nerve directly beneath it. A subluxation of L-2, which controls trophic supply into the acetabula socket, may compromise hip socket repair. L-5 supplies motor control around the hip. This is a scenario for rapid hip degeneration.

TWIST OF THE KNEE

Chronic pronation internally rotates the tibia on the femur and keeps the anterior horn of the medial meniscus directly under the medial femoral condyle. Failure to unload that area of the meniscus accelerates degenerative changes.

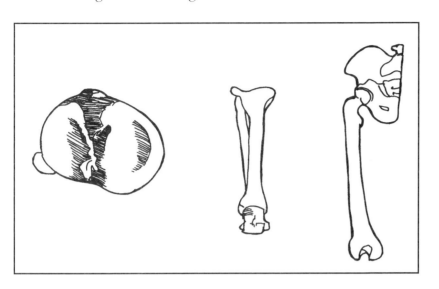

Pronation

Flattened Arch

HOW DOES THE FOOT CHANGE FROM ADDUCTION (SUPINATION) TO ABDUCTION (PRONATION) WHILE IN CONTACT WITH THE GROUND?

It all has to do with calcaneus relationship to the ground and the talus relationship to the calcaneus at an average angle of 45 degrees.

The talus head is more vertical in supination and it moves to horizontal in pronation while the calcaneus rocks from lateral tubercle to medial tubercle.

This moves the tibia obliquely across the foot as the talus falls medially.

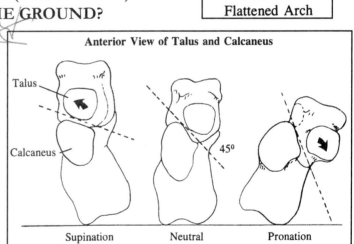

Anterior View of Talus and Calcaneus

Talus

Calcaneus

45°

Supination   Neutral   Pronation

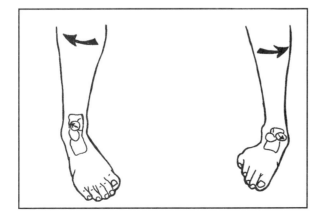

The tibia glides across on top of the talus from lateral to medial at an average angle of 45 degrees moving the ankle over the foot creating the appearance of forefoot deviation while the foot is still contacting the ground.

CHAPTER SEVEN

THE SECONDARY SHOCK ABSORBER OF THE BODY
KNEE FLEXION

At heel strike the knee is extended but must flex rapidly to absorb the shock associated with impact. The muscle that flexes the knee its first 15 degrees off of full extension is the popliteus. This is an internal rotator of the tibia which is supplied by the L-5 nerve root primarily.

If the foot is already in pronation at heel strike, which means the tibia may already be in internal rotation, can the popliteus muscle effectively flex the knee? Possibly not. Why?

The popliteus is an internal rotator and the tibia may be in maximum internal rotation.

(43, p. 151-153)

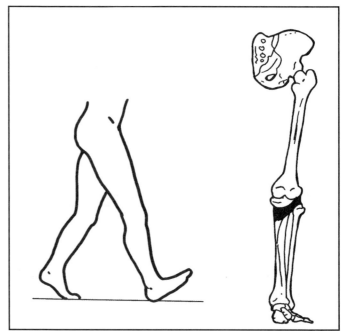

POSTERIOR TIBIAL MUSCLE FUNCTION

Normally the posterior tibia muscle contracts at heel strike. If the subtalar joint is already fully pronated or immobilized at heel strike, the posterior tibia muscle will exert all of its contraction force proximally instead of distally (reverses the origin and insertion), and will decelerate the tibia while the trunk and femur start to move over the implanted foot. Knee extension can be maintained and the knee may not flex to absorb shock.

Therefore adequate shock absorption may not occur at heel strike, unless subtalar joint pronation can occur to allow knee flexion.

Could a subluxation of L-5 or an L-4 disc protrusion affect knee flexion, the secondary shock absorber of the body ? Yes.

Could inadequate pronation and knee flexion transmit extra shock and create abnormal motion in the pelvis and lumbar spine ? Yes.

(43, p. 151-153)

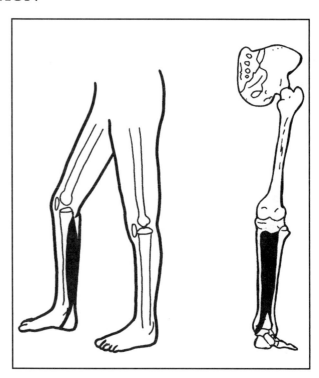

KNEE POSITION FOR DEGENERATIVE ARTHRITIS

Superior view of the Rt. knee

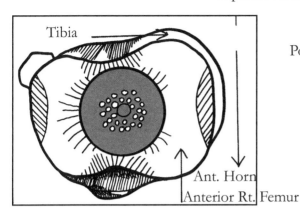

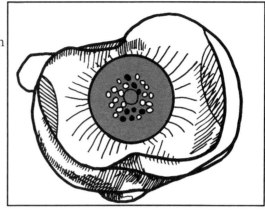

- **PRONATION**
- If the foot is stuck in pronation. Internal twisting of the tibia on the femur will result in maintaining constant pressure on the anterior horn of the medial meniscus. This leads to narrowing of the joint space and breaking down of the anterior medial meniscus.

- **SUPINATION**
- If the foot is stuck in supination. External twisting of the tibia on the femur will result in maintaining constant pressure on the posterior horn of the medial meniscus. This leads to narrowing of the joint space and breaking down of the posterior medial meniscus. This is much less common.

HERE IS WHAT AN EXPERT IN PODIATRY SAYS.

Quotable Quotes

1. "Any condition which prevents normal pronation of the subtalar joint results in pathologic shock. That shock is transmitted up the leg, into the pelvis, and on to the lumbar spine."
2. "This can lead to degenerate joint disease, muscle spasm, and chronic low back pain."
3. (Following an adjustment) "A functional orthoses which can re-establish some pronation at heel strike, will usually relieve back pain associated with faulty shock absorption."
(43, p. 153)

CHAPTER EIGHT

PHASES OF GAIT

The closer the foot, leg, thigh and pelvis approximates normal motion and position in time an degree, the better the prognosis for eliminating symptoms caused by abnormal motion or position.

Familiarity with normal motion and position of the foot, leg, thigh and pelvis during the gait cycle will enable the practitioner to appreciate the extent of malfunction when the pathologic gait occurs.

A gait cycle is defined as starting when the heel strikes the ground and ending after the swing phase has again found the same heel "striking".

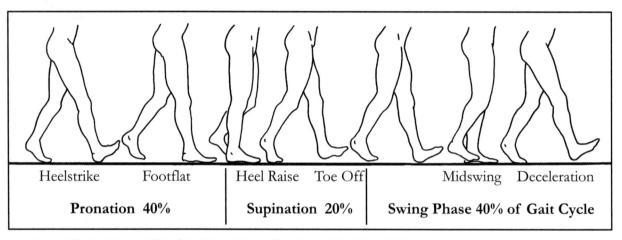

Heelstrike	Footflat	Heel Raise	Toe Off	Midswing	Deceleration
Pronation 40%		**Supination 20%**		**Swing Phase 40% of Gait Cycle**	

(5, p. 45-56; 25, p. 432-435; 43, p. 154-162; 45, p. 471, 516, 527)

STANCE/CONTACT - The period that the foot is in contact with the ground bearing weight. This is 62% of the full gait cycle.

SWING - That period when the foot is off of the ground being moved to another point of contact. This is 38% of the full gait cycle.

HEEL STRIKE - The moment the heel contacts the ground, until the forefoot makes contact with the ground.

MID STANCE - Following heel strike when the forefoot drops to fully contact the plantar surface of the foot with the ground (foot flat).

PUSH OFF/PROPULSIVE - When the heel lifts off of the ground until toe off occurs.

SINGLE SUPPORT - When only one foot contacts the ground. This occurs twice during a gait cycle.

DOUBLE SUPPORT - When both feet contact the ground. This occurs twice during a gait cycle.

STANCE / CONTACT PHASE OF GAIT – 62%

During the stance phase:

27% contact (HS to FF) heel strike to foot flat.

40% mid stance (FF to HR) foot flat to heel raise.

33% propulsion (HR to TO) heel raise to toe off.

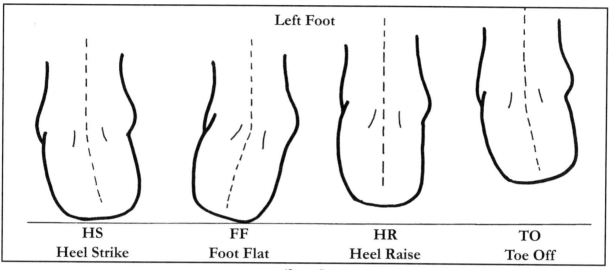

Left Foot

HS	FF	HR	TO
Heel Strike	Foot Flat	Heel Raise	Toe Off

(2, p. 6)

MIRROR IMAGE / GROUND REACTION FORCES

It can be helpful to view gait as if the patient is walking or running on a mirror. Ground reaction forces would be the reflection pushing back against the gravitational forces on the body at the same instant of contact.

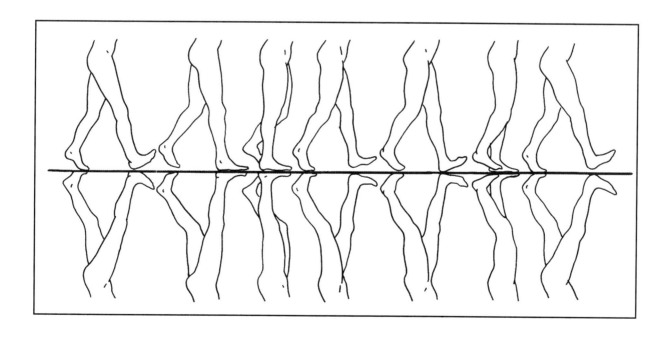

ACCELERATION / SWING LEG

Think of the contact leg as the stabilization leg preventing the body from crumpling to the earth from gravity drawing it downward.

Think of the swing leg as an accelerating mass moving forward that pulls the human frame forward as it reaches out ahead to advance to its next position of contact.

A jet engine not only creates thrust to push the plane forward but it also creates suction ahead of the engine to draw the engine into the vacuum.

PHASES OF GAIT ACCORDING TO HEARON

- Pronation begins at heel strike and ends at heel raise.
- Supination begins at heel raise and ends at toe off.
- When gait gets stuck in either of these positions the opposite function cannot occur and shock is no longer attenuated well.
- A full gait cycle is two steps ending with the same leg/foot forward that started forward.

PHASES OF GAIT ACCORDING TO HEARON

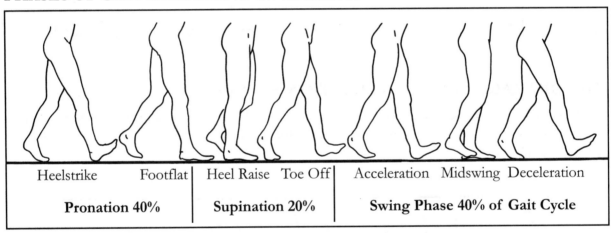

Heelstrike Footflat	Heel Raise Toe Off	Acceleration Midswing Deceleration
Pronation 40%	**Supination 20%**	**Swing Phase 40% of Gait Cycle**

I have had the privilege of having computerized gait analysis in the mid 1980's in my clinic measuring kilograms per square centimeter at 100th of a second on the sole of the feet during activities. It was the instrument used at the time by runners to determine the control factors of shoes and orthotics. I came up with this different view of 3 phases in the gait cycle which broke down the contact phase into two sections that I feel are important to identify.

GAIT LAB AND 3D SCANNER

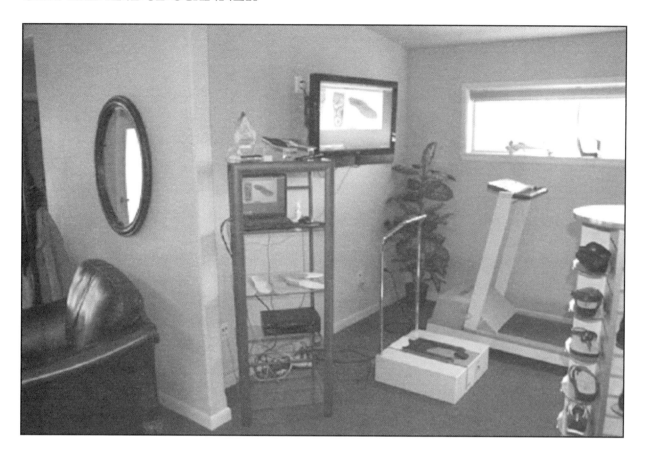

DIFFERENT DENSITY OPTIONS

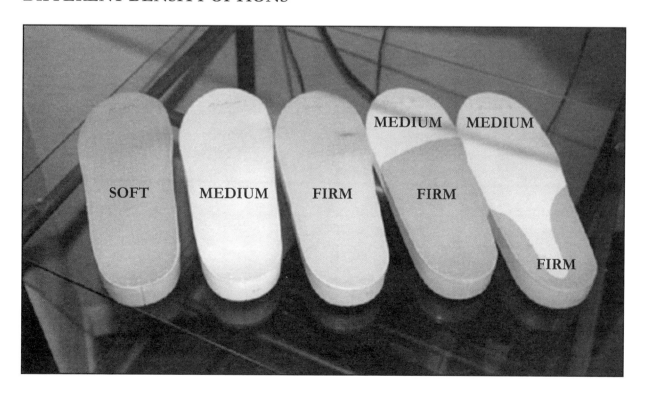

SOFT MEDIUM FIRM MEDIUM MEDIUM

FIRM FIRM

GAIT LAB AND 3D SCANNER

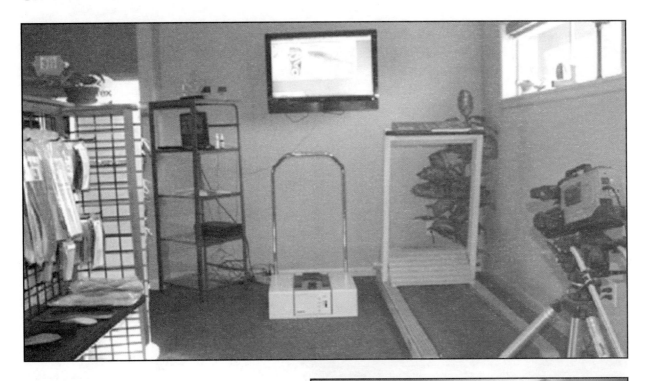

**REAL TIME FEEDBACK
FOR THE PATIENT
DURING GAIT**

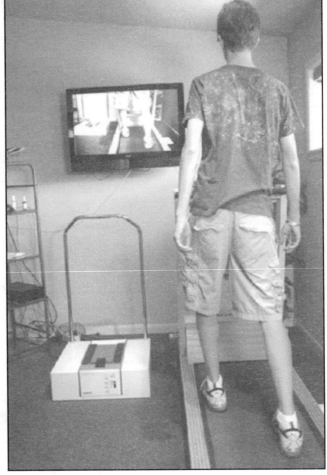

FEET EXAM STATION

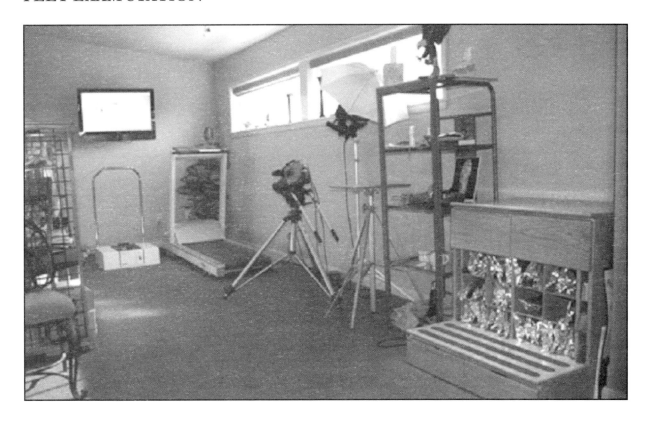

SOME TOOLS OF THE TRADE

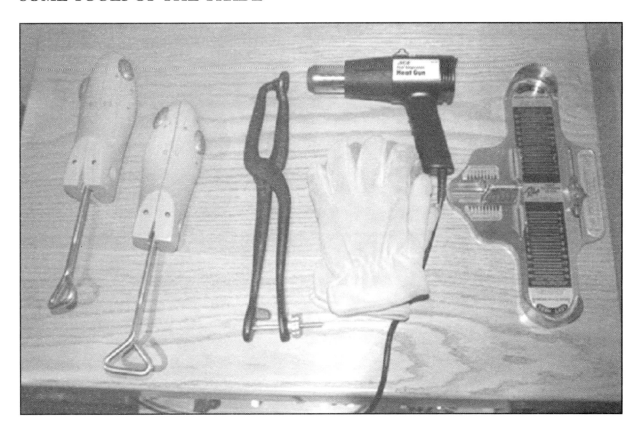

SHOES

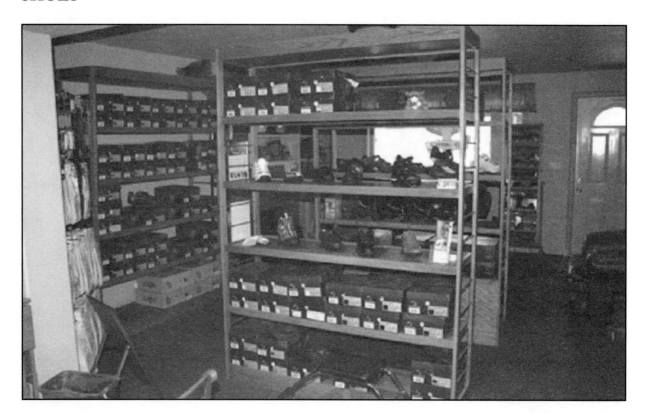

SANDALS

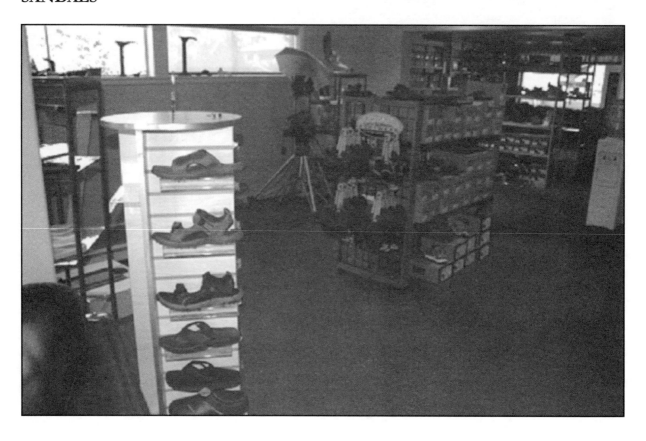

GENERIC ORTHOTICS

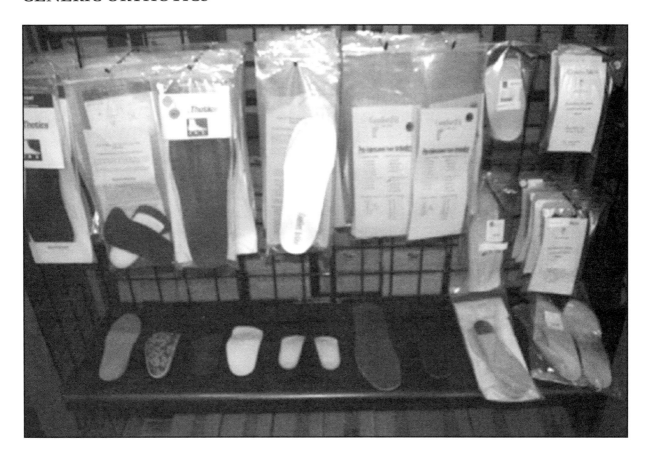

CHAPTER NINE

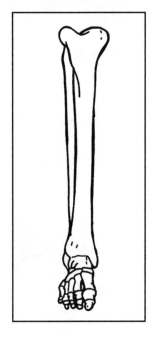

SHIN SPLINTS ACCORDING TO AMA

- ### SHIN SPLINTS: MEDIAL TIBIAL STRESS SYNDROME

The American Medical Association subcommittee report on the classification of sports injuries defines shin splints as discomfort and pain in the leg resulting from running repetitively on hard surfaces, or from forcible, excessive use of the foot dorsiflexors. The committee says that clinicians should limit the term "shin splints" to musculotendonous inflammations and exclude fractures and ischemic disorders.

(17, p. 105-113)

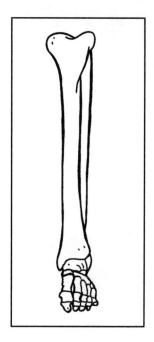

SHIN SPLINTS ACCORDING TO HEARON

- **ANTERIOR COMPARTMENT:** Is a muscular imbalance (10 to 1 ratio) between the gastroc-soleus and anterior tibia muscle. It happens during deceleration going down hill or at the end of a race while slowing down. Pressure along the lateral shin is painful.

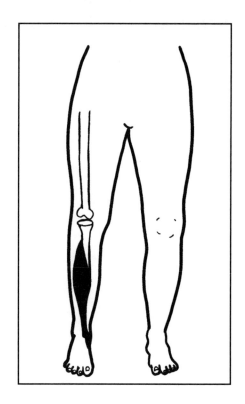

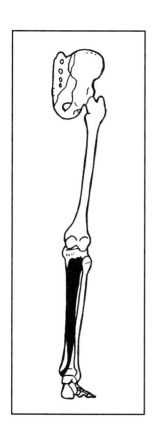

SHIN SPLINTS

- **POSTERIOR COM-PARTMENT:** Is from excessive pronation or from a fixated tarsal arch unable to supinate fully. This results in excess shock and pull at the origin of the posterior tibia muscle. It hurts to press along the medial side of the shin bone.

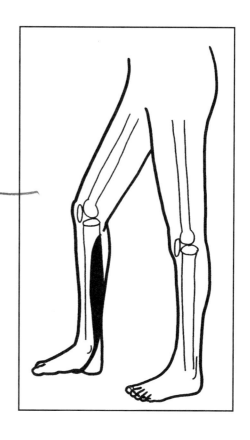

SHIN SPLINTS

The posterior tibia muscle is a plantar flexor of the foot. Medial Compartment Shin Splints are a direct result of excessive pronation and pulling of the posterior tibia muscle on the periosteum of the tibia. The origin and insertion reverses and thus pulls backward on the tibia. Control of pronation through foot orthotics fixes this condition usually.

Elastic compression of the entire shin from the ankle to the knee provides relief of symptoms usually. KGH

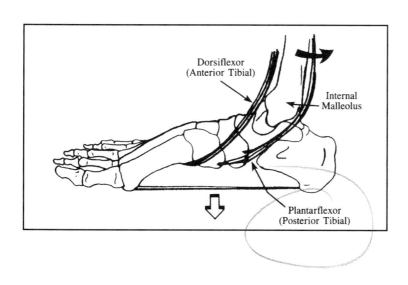

Dorsiflexor
(Anterior Tibial)

Internal
Malleolus

Plantarflexor
(Posterior Tibial)

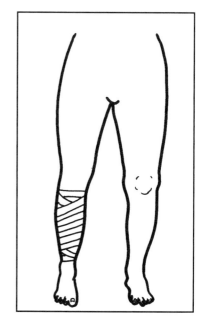

CHAPTER TEN

LAWS & AXIOMS OF HEALING

- PIEZOELECTRIC EFFECT.
- WOLFF'S LAW.
- DAVIS LAW.
- SHERRINGTON'S LAW.
- IF IT'S FIXATED MOBILIZE IT.
- IF IT'S HYPERMOBILE STABILIZE IT.
- ENERGY GOES WHERE ENERGY FLOWS.
- ENERGY STOPS WHERE ENERGY FLOPS.
- MECHANORECEPTOR RESPONSE.

PIEZOELECTRICITY FROM WIKIPEDIA
HTTP://EN.WIKIPEDIA.ORG/WIKI/PIEZOELECTRICITY. JULY 10, 2011

Piezoelectricity is **the ability of some materials** (notably crystals and certain ceramics, including bone) **to generate an electric potential in response to applied mechanical stress.** This may take the form of a separation of electrical charge across the crystal lattice. If the material is not short-circuited, the applied charge induces a voltage across the material. The word is derived from the Greek piezo or piezein, which means to squeeze or press.

- The piezoelectric effect is reversible in that materials exhibiting the direct piezoelectric effect (the production of an electric potential when stress is applied) also exhibit the reverse piezoelectric effect (the production of stress and/or strain when an electric field is applied). For example, lead zirconate titanate crystals will exhibit a maximum shape change of about 0.1% of the original dimension.

- The effect finds useful applications such as the production and detection of sound, generation of high voltages, electronic frequency generation, microbalances, and ultra fine focusing of optical assemblies. It is also the basis of a number of scientific instrumental techniques with atomic resolution and everyday uses such as acting as the ignition source for cigarette lighters and push-start propane barbeques.

WOLFF'S LAW FROM WIKIPEDIA
HTTP://EN.WIKIPEDIA.ORG/WIKI/WOLF'S_LAW. JULY 10, 2011

- Wolff's law is a theory developed by the German Anatomist/Surgeon Julius Wolff (1836-1902) in the 19th century that states that **bone** in a healthy person or animal **will adapt to the loads it is placed under**. If loading on a particular bone increases, the bone will remodel itself over time to become stronger to resist that sort of loading.

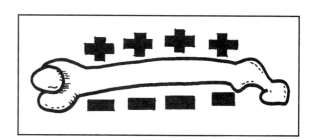

The external cortical portion of the bone becomes thicker as a result. The converse is true as well: if the loading on a bone decreases, the bone will become weaker due to turnover, it is less metabolically costly to maintain and there is no stimulus for continued remodeling that is required to maintain bone mass.[

DAVIS' LAW FROM WIKIPEDIA
HTTP://EN.WIKIPEDIA.ORG/WIKI/DAVIS%27_LAW. JULY 10,2011

- Davis' Law is used in anatomy to describe how **soft tissue models along imposed demands**. It is the corollary to Wolff's law. It is used in part to describe muscle-length relationships and to predict rehabilitation and postural distortion treatments as far as muscle length is concerned.
- This is not necessarily describing myohypertrophy (muscle growth) the shortening of muscle in response to resistance but it explains also how a muscle will lengthen in response to stretching.
- Because most major muscles have an opposite, the protagonistic and antagonistic muscles (and their related synergistic and groups of muscles) will end up reciprocating each other's length. A strong and inflexible gastro soleus complex (calf) will therefore result in a weak and flexible tibialis anterior (shin muscle).
- References: Nutt, John Joseph, Diseases and deformities of the foot. New York: E. B. Treat & Co.; 1915, pp. 157-158. (Out of copyright. Available as a pdf in total via Google books).
- Spencer AM, Practical podiatric orthopedic procedures. Cleveland: Ohio College of Podiatric Medicine; 1978.
- Tippett, Steven R. and Michael L. Voight, Functional Progression for Sport Rehabilitation. Champaigne IL: Human Kinetics; 1995, ISBN 0-873-22660-7, p. 4.

IN REVIEW THESE LAWS STATE THESE 3 THINGS.

- The ability of material to generate an electric potential in response to applied mechanical stress
- Bone will adapt to the loads it is placed under..
- Soft tissue models along imposed demands.

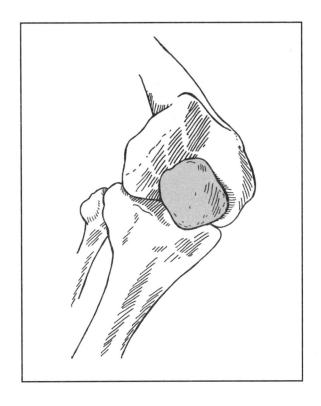

THEREFORE TISSUE HEALS AND ADAPTS THROUGH POLARITY GENERATED BY LOAD AND MOTION.

The ligament poles sense their direction and align the fibers to reconnect one fragile fiber at a time until the whole ligament is complete.

This process can take up to three months to complete the healing.

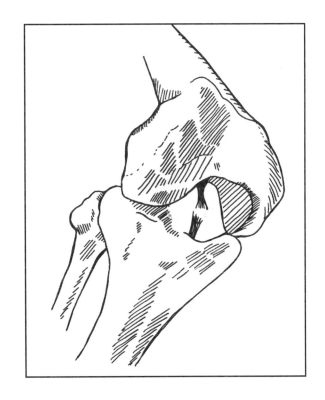

THE NUMBER ONE PROBLEM THAT GETS IN THE WAY OF THIS HEALING IS: DOCTORS

Doctors are taught to perform objective tests on patients each visit (like an anterior drawer test) to justify their procedures and treatment plan. They follow the SOAP format – Subjective, Objective, Assessment, Plan.

Doctors tear these fragile fibers unwittingly doing these tests repetitively and therefore believe they don't heal.

(31, 44)

ANTERIOR DRAWERS TEST TEARS FRAGILE NEW FIBERS.

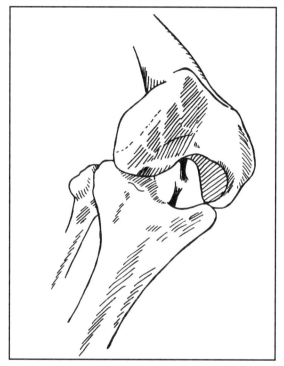 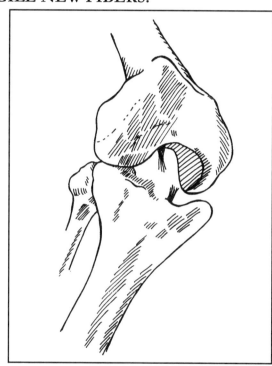

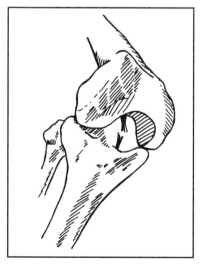 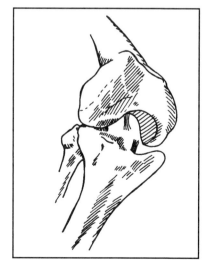 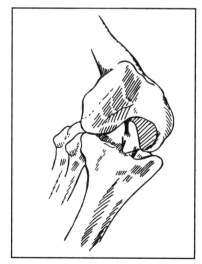

(31, 44)

PROPER PROTOCOL FOR LIGAMENTS
THIS IS THE APPLICATION OF THE LAWS OF HEALING.

Adjust the joint to restore normal relationship so the tissues heal in the normal tight position instead of a stretched and elongated ligament position.

Stabilize the joint with taping, supports or bracing to prevent it from moving out of its normal physiologic envelope.

Allow motion through the non-painful range of motion which stimulates the polarity for the tissues to heal in the correct direction.

SHERRINGTON'S LAW

The relationship between weak and tight muscles is reciprocal and produces inhibition equally as well as excitation on opposite sides. When this is out of balance, one method is to find the inhibition and adjust to correct it. Another approach is to stretch and or relax the strong muscle. However you may activate the weak muscle to get the tight muscle to relax. All have functional uses in rehabilitation.

(7)
Dynamic Chiropractic – March 26, 2010, Vol. 28, Issue 07
Muscle Imbalance: The Goodheart and Janda Models
By Scott Cuthbert, BA, DC, BCAO

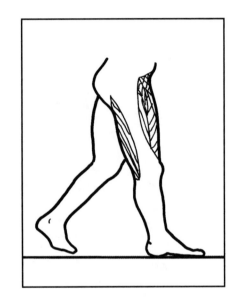

IF IT'S FIXATED MOBILIZE IT.

- A fixated joint has limited motion and does not glide through it's normal physiologic envelope.
- This may be due to joint adhesions or mechanoreceptor inhibition of adjacent muscles.
- Adjustments (manipulation) frequently will restore motion and mobility. Joints need to glide to adapt to shapes, terrain and position in space. These functions allow us to accommodate to uneven surfaces as well as absorb shock and share load over a joints surface. Muscles also need range of motion to function through full contraction and relaxation which acts as either a force transmitter or absorber.

IF IT'S HYPERMOBILE STABILIZE IT

- A hypermobile joint has excess motion outside of it's normal physiologic envelope. Joints that exceed their normal physiologic envelope and travel beyond their set boundaries tend to damage more tissue. This sets up compensatory reactions above and below the joint. What healing that does take place is usually elongated and unable to contain joint glide within safe limits.
- This may be due to trauma or long term stretching (plastic deformation) of the ligaments in the joint that have healed at a pathological length.
- Stabilizing the joint with taping, supports, bracing or foot orthotics within its normal motion is essential. The purpose of using supports is to contain the joint with in normal limits while allowing tissue to heal at normal lengths.

ENERGY GOES WHERE ENERGY FLOWS

- Where there is stress/friction over time there is a build up of tissue. (e.g. Calluses, increased bone mass or growth, increased muscle mass). The human body tells a story about how it uses energy and it is very observable much of the time. Where the body is trim it is probably being used a lot. Where there is excess fat or less tone it probably is not being used as much. Friction on the body will create calluses and the more friction applied will usually create heavier calluses. This can be easily observed on the bottom of the feet and palpated for differences of thickness.

ENERGY STOPS WHERE ENERGY FLOPS.

- Where there is no stress/friction over time there is a lack of build up of tissue, (eg. Baby skin, decreased bone mass and muscle mass, fat deposits).
- Take a look at yourself and check out where the fat is. How much do you exercise that area? Energy is stopping and flopping there.
- Baby like skin on the foot is probably not getting much friction.

"IF YOU SHOW ME A WAY TO IRRITATE THE PERIOSTEUM, I'LL SHOW YOU A WAY TO GROW BONE." (DR. RUSSELL ERHARDT CIRCA-1976)

- Just look at a calcaneal heel spur being tugged on by the plantar fascia at the medial tubercle.
- A big toe bunion is another example.
- Buttressing at the anterior talar dome from irritation by the anterior tibial ridge.

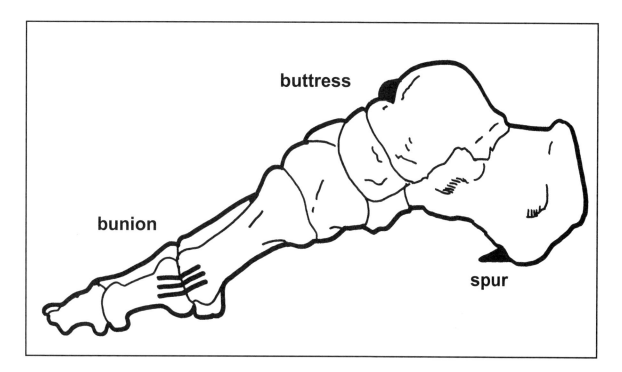

CHAPTER ELEVEN

ANKLE MORTISE

The medial and lateral malleoli viewed from above reveals a postero-lateral angled transverse plane. The medial malleolus extends 1/3 of the way down the medial talus. The lateral malleolus extends down the length of the entire lateral talus.

The body of the talus is a wedge shaped bone with the wider portion anterior. Upon dorsiflexion the wider portion spreads the malleoli like a wedge between them. This results in the fibula moving laterally tightening the inter osseous ligaments and helps to stabilize the ankle.

Plantar flexion of the talus is more unstable in the ankle mortise due to laxity of the inter osseous ligaments when the narrow portion of the talus is engaged.

(5, p. 1-3; 33, p. 28-41; 42, p. 459-471)

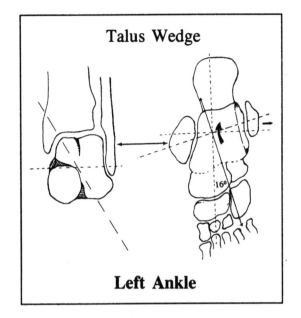

Talus Wedge

Left Ankle

The interosseous ligament extends from the inner aspect of the tibia inferiorly and laterally to the inner aspect of the fibula.

During dorsiflexion, the wedge of the talus widens the mortise laterally, forcing the fibula to rise slightly allowing these fibers to become more nearly horizontal.

Plantar flexion, on the other hand, slackens this ligament and allows the fibula to lower itself.

The anterior tibiofibular ligament runs parallel to the interosseous ligament and reinforces it.

The posterior tibiofibular ligament runs parallel to the interosseous ligament and reinforces it.

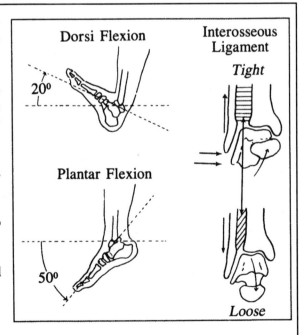

Dorsi Flexion

20°

Plantar Flexion

50°

Interosseous Ligament

Tight

Loose

LIGAMENTS

The lateral collateral ligaments have three bands that give the ankle joint support. They are;

    A. Anterior Talofibular -   from the neck of the talus to the tip of the fibula.
    B. Calcaneofibular   -   from the calcaneus to the tip of the fibula.
    C. Posterior Talofibular -   from the body of the talus to the tip of the fibula.

Note: The most frequently injured ligaments during an ankle sprain are the anterior talofibular and the calcaneofibular. This is usually an inversion injury while the ankle is in plantar flexion, which is the most unstable position for the ankle.

The deltoid ligaments are four bands that support the medial portion of the ankle joint from the medial malleolus to the navicular, the sustentaculum talus, and the posterior aspect of the talus.

    A. Tibionavicular
    B. Anterior Talotibial
    C. Calcaneotibial
    D. Posterior Talotibial

Note: An avulsion of the malleolus is more likely than a tear of the deltoid ligament during severe eversion sprain because of its strength.

Note: The talus is the only bone in the foot without any tendons attaching to it.

(5, p.3-8; 32, p. 90-92; 42, p. 459-471)

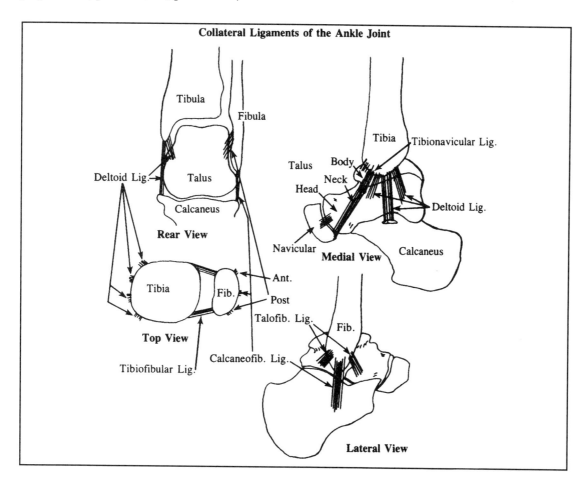

41

X-RAYS OF THE ANKLE

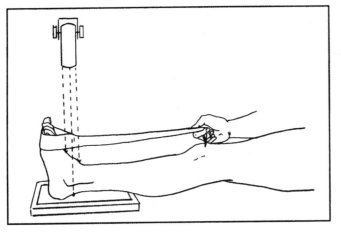

Anteroposterior Ankle Projection

Film Size   10 x 12 inches (24 x 30 cm)

Central Ray   Center between the malleoli.

Medial Oblique Ankle Projection

Film Size   1/2 of a 10 x 12 inches (24 x 30 cm) *Use the other half for the A-P Projection.*

Central Ray   Center between the malleoli with the foot internally rotated 35-45 degrees.

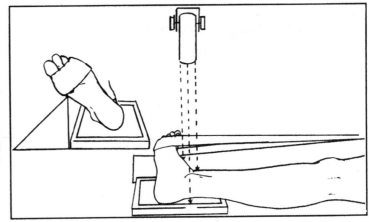

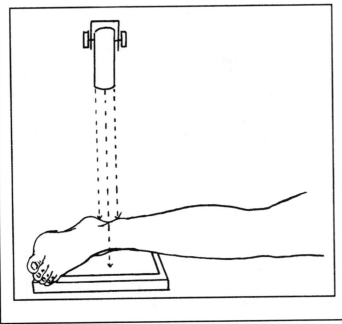

Lateral Ankle Projection

Film Size   8 x 10 inches (18 x 24 cm)

Central Ray   Center of medial malleolus.

ORTHOPEDIC TESTS OF THE ANKLE AND FOOT

ANTERIOR FOOT DRAW

Stabilize the anterior distal tibia with one hand. Then grasp the posterior calcaneus with the other hand and pull it anterior. Normally there is no movement of the foot anteriorly in the ankle mortise. If movement occurs, it is indicative of an anterior talofibular ligament instability that is secondary to its rupture.

(33, p. 215)

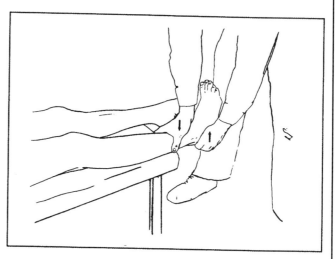

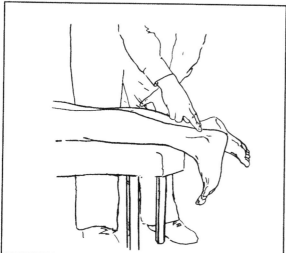

HOFFA'S SIGN

The patient is prone, with their feet hanging well over the end of the table. Observe for increased dorsiflexion of one foot and palpate the achilles tendon on that side to feel if it is less taut than the other side. If present, it is indicative of an avulsion fracture of the calcaneus. A fragment may be seen or felt behind either malleolus.

(33, p.287)

HOMAN'S SIGN

With the patient supine and the legs fully extended, you firmly dorsiflex the foot on the ankle. If the patient experiences well localized deep pain in the back of the calf or behind the knee, it is indicative of thrombophlebitis (thrombosis of the deep veins of the leg).

(33, p.287)

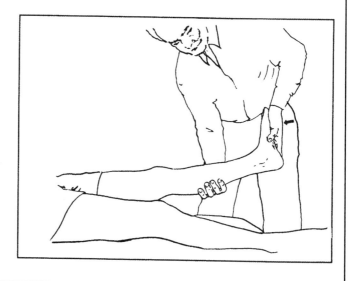

METATARSALGIA

Press the outer four toes into dorsiflexion and percuss the metatarsal heads with a reflex hammer. If neuritic type pain occurs, it is indicative of anterior metatarsalgia due to inflammation of the metatarsophalangeal joints.

(33, p.326)

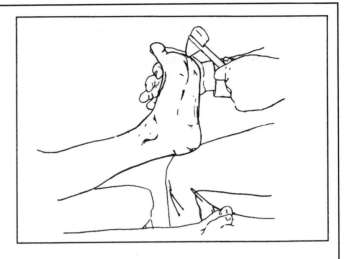

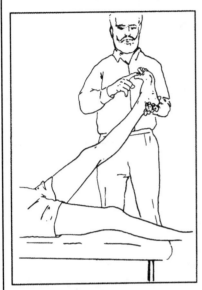

SICARD'S SIGN

Similar to the Lasegue (straight leg raise) test, the patients leg is raised just short of producing pain. If sciatic pain is produced when you dorsiflex the big toe it is indicative of a sciatic radiculopathy.

(33, p. 326, 356)

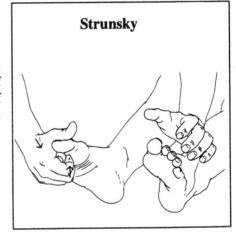

Strunsky

STRUNSKY'S SIGN

The examiner grasps the patients lateral four toes and suddenly flexes them. This is painless in a normal foot. If lancinating pain occurs, the sign is present. This is indicative of a drop of the metatarsal arch with resultant metatarsophalangeal inflammation.

(33, p.362)

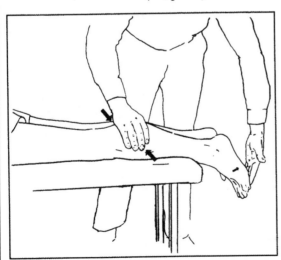

THOMPSONS

With the patient prone and their feet hanging over the end of the table, squeeze the calf below its widest portion and observe for plantar flexion of the foot. If this does not occur, it is indicative of a complete rupture of the achilles tendon.

(33, p. 362, 366)

NEUTRAL POSITION OF THE FOOT/SUBTALAR JOINT (S.T.J.) NEUTRAL POSITION

The position where the S.T.J. is neither pronated nor supinated. When the S.T.J. is in neutral position, **there is a congruency of the talonavicular joint**. This can be palpated at the joint articulation between the head of the talus and the navicular.

(43, p. 154-157)

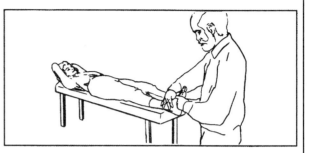

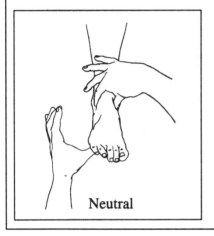

Neutral

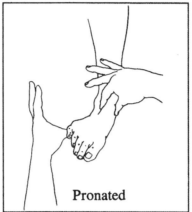

Pronated

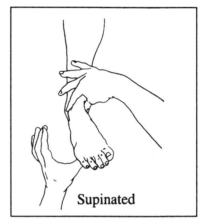

Supinated

NEUTRAL POSITION

- When the foot is neither dorsiflexed or plantar flexed, adducted or abducted, inverted or everted. It is none of these. It is neutral.
- When the foot is in neutral position there is a congruency of the talo-navicular joint. There are equal indentations on each side of the joint.
- At this time a perpendicular to the shaft of the tibia is taken down to the metatarsal heads and the angle is measured. This is the approach angle of the foot to the ground.
- Normal range is between 0 to 4-6 degrees varus.

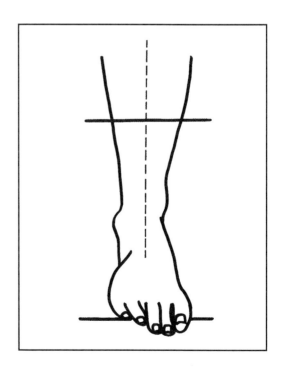

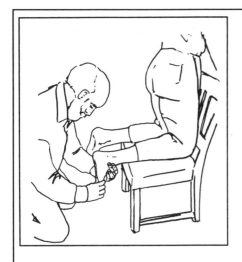

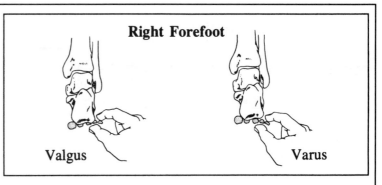

Right Forefoot

Valgus　　　　　　　　　　　Varus

Note: To successfully attain neutral position, it is important to lock the midfoot against the rearfoot by pressing the 4th and 5th metatarsal heads into dorsiflexion. This will fully pronate the midtarsal joint and allow correct viewing of varus and valgus deformities when the foot is held in neutral position.

(43, p. 154-157)

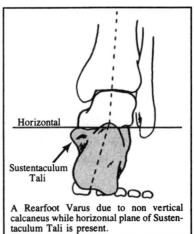

Horizontal

Sustentaculum Tali

A Rearfoot Varus due to non vertical calcaneus while horizontal plane of Sustentaculum Tali is present.

FOREFOOT MEASURING DEVICE (FFMD)

FFMD when applied correctly to the foot gives accurate angles of the forefoot.

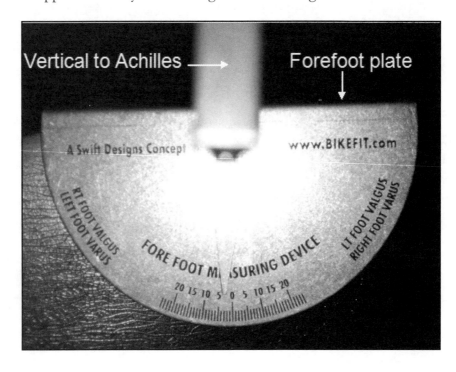

Vertical to Achilles　　　　　Forefoot plate

A Swift Designs Concept　　　www.BIKEFIT.com

RT FOOT VALGUS
LEFT FOOT VARUS

FORE FOOT MEASURING DEVICE

LT FOOT VALGUS
RIGHT FOOT VARUS

20 15 10 5 0 5 10 15 20

FFMD

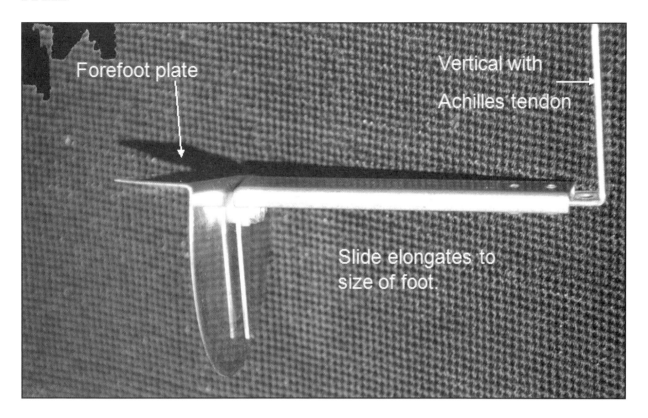

APPLICATION OF FFMD

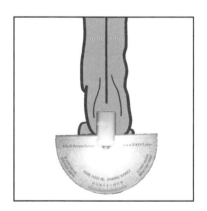 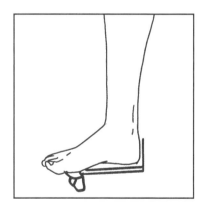 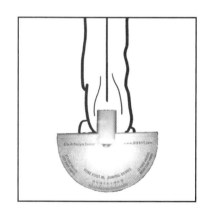

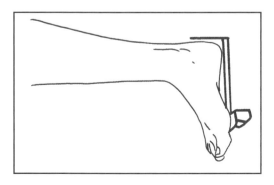

The forefoot-rearfoot frontal plane relationship was tested with a forefoot measuring device and a goniometer. Of the 234 measured feet, 86.67% had a varus, 8.75% had a valgus, and 4.58% had a neutral forefoot-rearfoot relationship.

(15)

(J Orthop Sports Phys Ther. 1994 Oct;20(4):200-6.)

Garbalosa JC, McClure MH, Catlin PA, Wooden M

SUBLUXATION OF THE TALUS:

The talus typically moves anterior during an ankle sprain, which results in limited dorsiflexion of the ankle due to jamming of the condyle against the anterior tibial ridge. Document the distance of difference in dorsiflexion (e.g. 1/4", 1/2", 1", 5mm, 10mm, 15mm, etc.).

Eighty percent of all ankle sprains are inversion sprains, in which the talus gets rotated medially, creating a false or exaggerated forefoot varus deformity. In the event of a eversion sprain, the talus rotates laterally at its head and creates a false or exaggerated forefoot valgus. Document the angles of varus or valgus before the adjustment (e.g. 7 degrees, 12 degrees, 15 degrees, etc.).

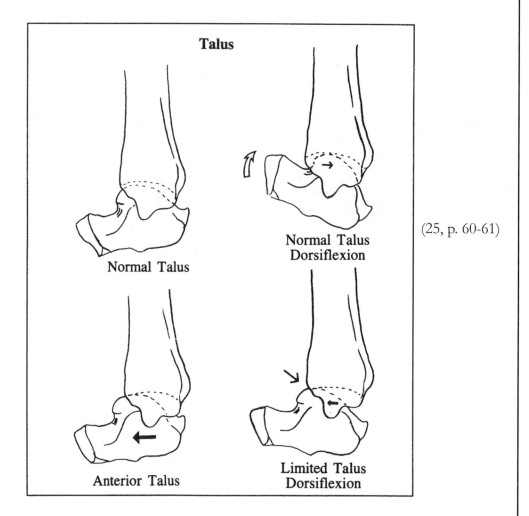

(25, p. 60-61)

This is exactly why it is so important to check for this subluxation before casting a foot in the neutral position. The neutral position may be pathomechanical and so will be the foot orthotic if one is made without correcting the talus subluxation.

It is important to note at this time that not all forefoot varus or valgus conditions are a result of subluxations of the foot. You cannot adjust out what God made that way and expect it to perform well. If all of the talus signs are negative, then neutral position is probably correct.

SIGNS

- Limited firm dorsiflexion of involved foot.
- Anterior fossa is shallow, being filled by the talus.
- While holding the foot in the neutral position, it will be evident that the head of the talus is either medial or lateral, because the foot is definitely not centered.
- Limited movement of fibular head at the knee upon ankle dorsiflexion.
- Pain on side of injury when palpated if acute.

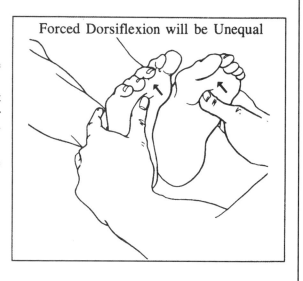

Forced Dorsiflexion will be Unequal

The feet are firmly dorsiflexed to the end range of motion in the joint while the malleoli are even. Compare the 1st MTP joints with each other. They should be even.

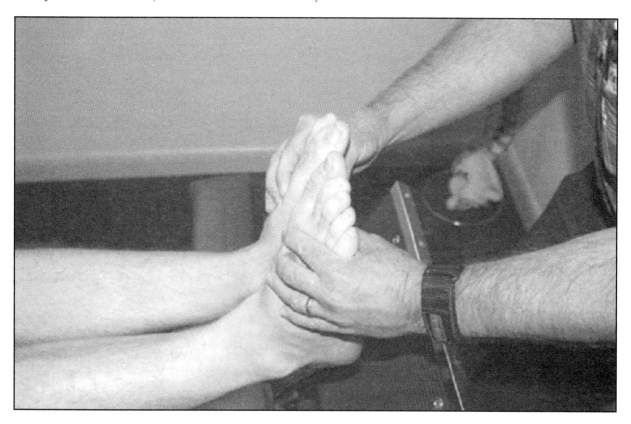

49

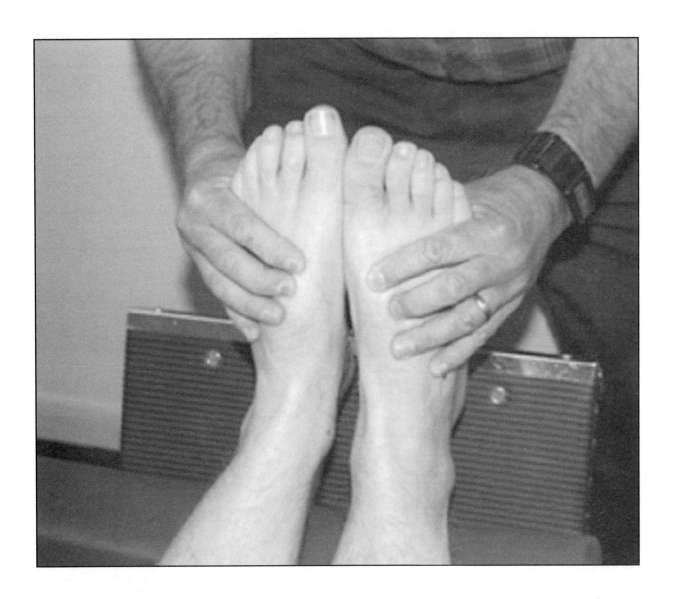

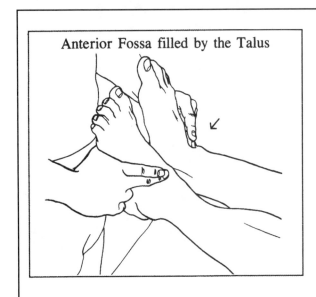

Anterior Fossa filled by the Talus

MUSCLE AFFECTED

The talus is the only bone in the foot with no muscles and tendons attaching to it.

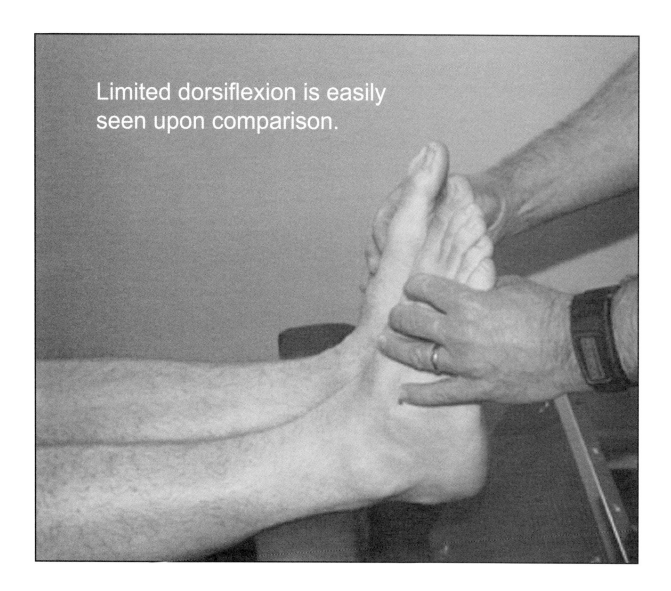

Limited dorsiflexion is easily seen upon comparison.

What other doctors frequently interpret the dorsiflexion difference of the feet to is a "short Achilles tendon" or a "tight gastrocnemius/soleus complex" or an "equines foot.

So I ask them "if that is true then an adjustment of the ankle won't change that position – is that correct?" And they say "Yes".

I then adjust the ankle and demonstrate with them how the feet have become even.

They typically take about three demonstrations before they can believe their eyes and hands checking the feet pre and post adjustment.

51

ADJUSTMENTS OF THE TALUS:

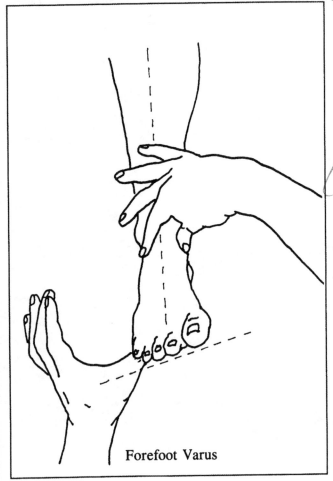

Forefoot Varus

ANTERO-MEDIAL TALUS:

SIGNS

- Limited firm dorsiflexion of the foot.
- Shallow anterior talar fossa to palpation.
- Varus forefoot that becomes more normal following the talus adjustment.

IMPACT OF INJURY

Inversion ankle sprains; plantar flexion and inversion of the foot while coming down on the involved limb.

CONTACT

Stand facing the knees of a prone patient on the opposite side of the involved leg. Flex the involved leg to 90 degrees and place your knee closest to the head across the lower hamstrings of both legs with equal pressure. Using the hand closest to the head, grasp the lateral ankle like a pistol grip with your middle finger on the mid talar fossa as the contact finger, and your thumb around the Achilles tendon.

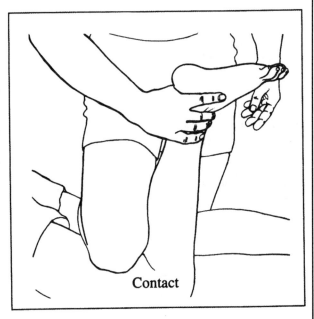

Contact

STABILIZATION

The hand toward the feet is for stabilization, and is used to support the contact finger and thumb while lifting the inside of the foot before the thrust until you feel distraction of the joint.

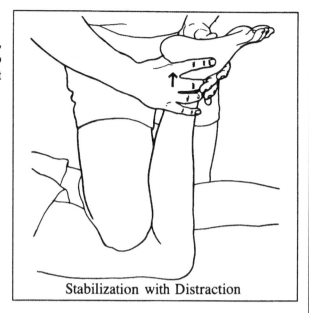

Stabilization with Distraction

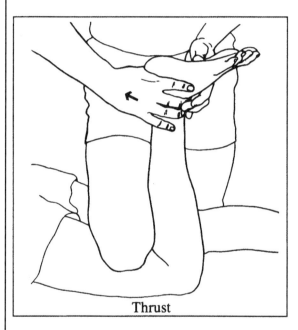

Thrust

THRUST

After applying the stabilization hand, lift the ankle toward the ceiling until you feel distraction. Thrust the talus straight back toward the heel. Rotation is taken care of automatically by your position.

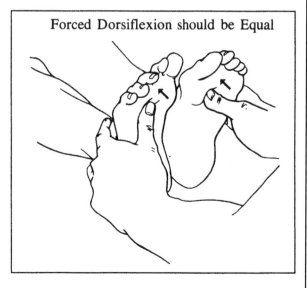

Forced Dorsiflexion should be Equal

POST CHECKS

Is foot dorsiflexion now even or much closer to even ?

Are both anterior talar fossas equal in depth ?

Is the forefoot varus decreased or absent? By how much? Please document these findings.

ANTERO-LATERAL TALUS:

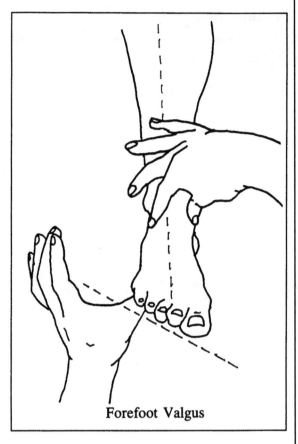

Forefoot Valgus

SIGNS

Limited firm dorsiflexion of the foot. Shallow anterior talar fossa. Forefoot valgus that becomes normal or significantly improved following the talus adjustment.

IMPACT OF INJURY

Eversion ankle sprains; plantar flexion and eversion of the foot while landing on the involved limb.

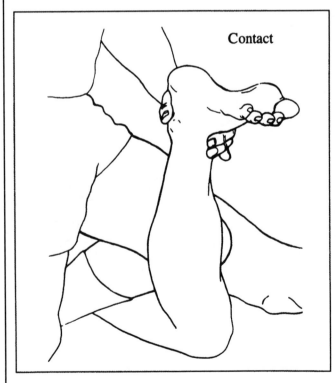

Contact

CONTACT

Stand facing the knees of a prone patient on the same side of involvement. Flex the involved leg to 90 degrees and place your knee closest to the head across the hamstrings of only the involved leg. Using the hand closest to the head, grasp the medial ankle like a pistol grip with your middle finger on the mid talar fossa and your thumb around the Achilles tendon.

STABILIZATION

The hand toward the feet is the stabilization hand, and is used to support the contact finger with its middle finger. The thumb can either go over the cuboid or around the Achilles tendon.

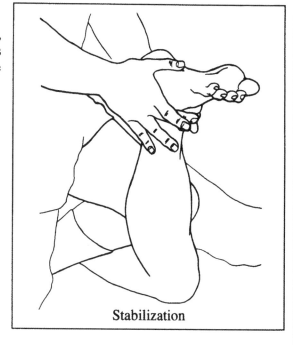

Stabilization

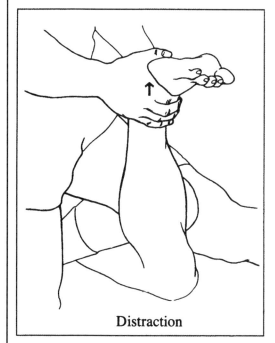

Distraction

Apply the stabilization hand and lift the ankle until you feel distraction.

THRUST

Thrust the talus straight back toward the heel. Rotation is taken care of by your position automatically.

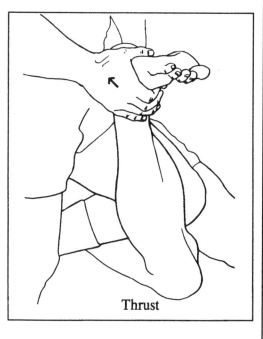

Thrust

POST CHECKS

Do the dorsiflexion press test to see if both feet dorsiflex evenly and check the depth of the anterior talar fossa. Note the change of the forefoot valgus, then document your findings.

TARSAL TUNNEL SYNDROME/POSTERIOR TIBIAL NERVE SYNDROME (18,p. 100; 54,p. 15)

SIGNS

Numbness about the medial malleolus (the inside of the ankle) and medial plantar aspect of the foot. This may wake the patient up in the middle of the night and require motion of the joint or massage to relieve the symptoms.

IMPACT OF INJURY

Cramping and compression of the calf. Repetitive motions that force the heel and forefoot into the valgus position, which tightens the flexor retinaculum and the abductor hallucis, thereby compressing the nerve. This compression neuropathy is similar to carpal tunnel syndrome in the hand. It is for this reason that I am moved to call this the *Tarsal Flat Syndrome*, because the valgus position of the foot usually flattens the tarsal arch.

LOCATION OF NERVE

Behind the medial malleolus, palpate the posterior tibial pulse. The posterior tibial nerve is one finger breadth behind this.

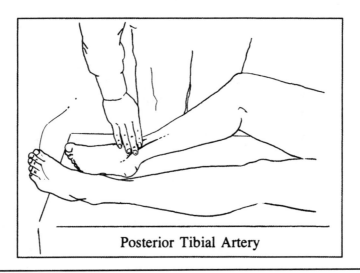

Posterior Tibial Artery

ORTHOPEDIC TEST - *TINEL TAP*

When tapping on the posterior tibial nerve, a positive test will elicit pain along the nerve into the medial foot.

TREATMENT

Correction of valgus stresses into the rearfoot and forefoot should be the first approach at reducing compression of the retinaculum on the posterior tibial nerve. Correction may be as simple as wearing a shoe with a strong heel counter or a good tarsal arch support. The probability of the need for correction of foot subluxations and a foot orthotic is high for a person with this problem. Lodye taping of the foot with Zonas Porous tape or a foot slipper with a heel lock made with elastic tape can give temporary relief, until a permanent resolution is produced.

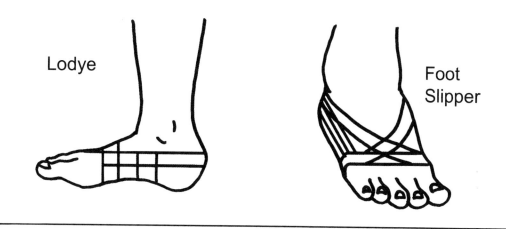

Lodye

Foot Slipper

CHAPTER TWELVE

The Foot
(5, p.1-3; 43, p.28-41; 56, p.459-471)

ANATOMY OF THE FOOT: There are twenty six bones of the foot that may be divided into seven tarsals, five metatarsals and fourteen phalanges.

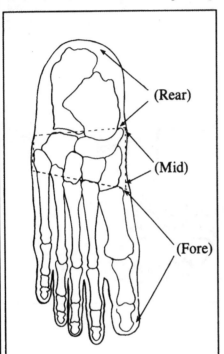

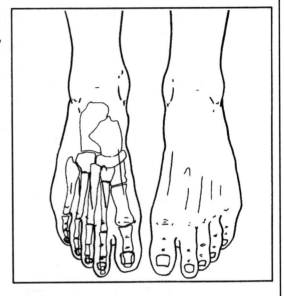

Functionally speaking the foot has five major segments.
1. The rear foot
2. The middle medial
3. The middle lateral
4. The medial forefoot
5. The lateral forefoot

THE REAR FOOT

A posterior segment that is under the tibia and supports it which includes the talus and calcaneus. The talus is a domed wedge shaped bone in the ankle joint with the wide portion of the dome at the anterior aspect. Its medial side is in the sagittal plane. Its lateral side is oblique to the sagittal plane. It is responsible for medial foot motion during pronation and supination. It is the keystone of the medial longitudinal tarsal arch.

The calcaneus is under and behind the talus, supporting it and controlling it during the pronation and supination process. It is responsible for lateral foot motion during pronation and supination.

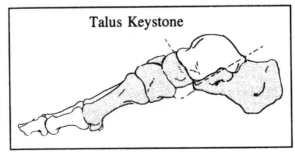
Talus Keystone

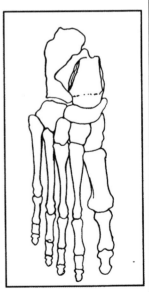

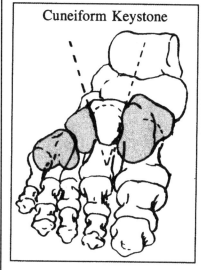

Cuneiform Keystone

THE MID FOOT (56, p.469)

The middle medial segment is a continuation of the medial foot from the talus. It proceeds distally to the navicular, which then articulates with the three cuneiforms, the first, second and third. Together, these three cuneiforms, with the medial three metatarsals, make up the medial three rays with phalanges. It is important to note at this time that the middle or second cuneiform is the keystone of the transverse arch of the medial mid foot.

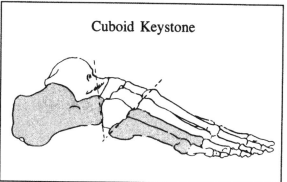

Cuboid Keystone

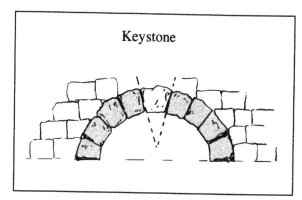

Keystone

The middle lateral segment is a continuation of the lateral foot from the calcaneus. It is the cuboid bone, which is a wedge shaped bone with the wide part facing medially articulating with the navicular and lateral cuneiform. It also articulates with the base for the 4th and 5th rays of metatarsal phalangeal segments. It should be noted that the cuboid is the keystone of the lateral longitudinal arch of the foot.

THE FOREFOOT

The medial forefoot consists of the medial three metatarsals and phalanges. Each series of bones are called rays. Each one articulates proximally with the corresponding three cuneiforms.

The lateral forefoot consists of the lateral two metatarsals, and the 4th and 5th phalanges. These two lateral rays articulate proximally with the cuboid.

Of course the medial and lateral foot articulate to tie the units together to form what is commonly thought to be a single unit biomechanically. However, it seems to function at times in a separate way. More like a medial and lateral foot than the classic rear, middle and forefoot. However these latter classifications do apply to the medial and lateral sides individually.

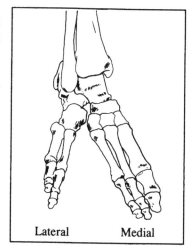

Lateral   Medial

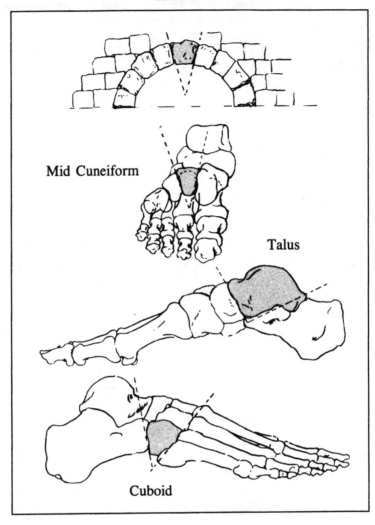

Mid Cuneiform

Talus

Cuboid

FOOT PRONATION

Foot Pronation is the primary shock absorber of the body.

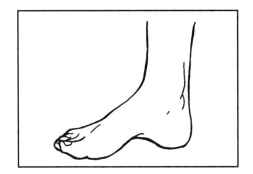

Normal feet should pronate with weight-bearing by slowing down the drop of the arch to the ground (known as eccentric contraction of the posterior tibia muscle).

Pronation thus absorbs shock by attenuating the impact of ground contact.

Motion must occur at the mid tarsal joints for successful pronation to function well.

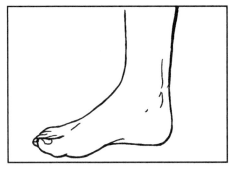

Pronation of the foot as measured by the navicular drop test is about 10 mm. This navicular drop elongates the foot lengthwise increasing surface area and tightening the plantar fascia. Nine to eleven mm is considered within normal excursion. Fifteen mm of navicular drop is outside of normal limits and requires correction.

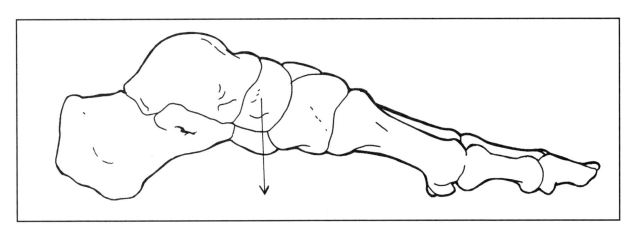

If there is that much drop I would suspect a hypermobile foot that needs stabilization due to plastic deformation of the ligaments. This is where a more rigid orthotic is useful for a period of three to six months to allow shortening of the ligaments and strengthening of the foot muscles.

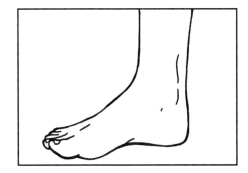

What most people don't realize is that it is not usually a matter of excessive drop.

It is more often a matter of recovering from a fixated foot stuck in pronation and unable to supinate fully again.

Most feet are stuck in the down (pronated) position and can't return to the raised arch (supinated) position.

To determine the difference it is necessary to perform joint glide tests of the feet.

FOOT JOINT GLIDE

Checking glide of the first met base and first cuneiform by shearing the joint through its plane line.

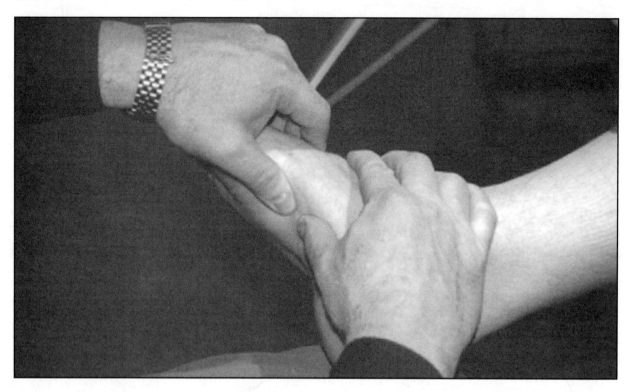

Notice the skin wrinkles from normal joint glide. You and the patient can readily see and feel this motion. A fixated joint will not move like this and is usually tender to test. A hypermobile joint will exceed this motion. Joint glide can be done on most joints of the feet.

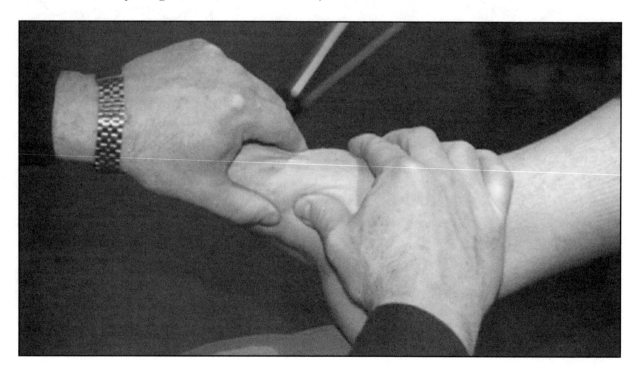

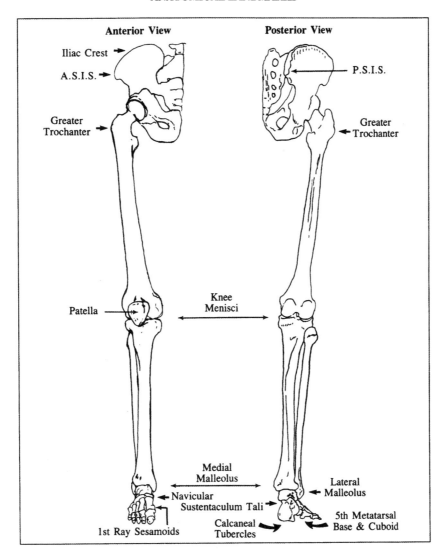

Breakdown of the medial longitudinal tarsal arch from
   excess pronation usually results in a cascading
   sequence of events that will usually develop into one
   or more of the following anomalies;

    Big toe bunion
    Calcaneal heel spur
    Plantar fasciitis
    Posterior compartment shin splints
    Patellar tracking syndrome
    Sacroiliac fixation or hypermobility
    Hip degenerative arthritis
    Facet jamming
    Disc herniation or prolapse with no history of trauma
    Unstable lumbar spine and sometimes pelvis

Correction of foot pronation through restoration of motion and glide in the tarsals by manipulation of the fixated bones in each foot will restore normal excursion of the arches and improve shock absorption. A functional foot orthotic will maintain arch excursion and joint mobility within normal limits and can stabilize a hypermobile foot.

POSITION FIXATIONS OF THE FOOT: (2,p.2)

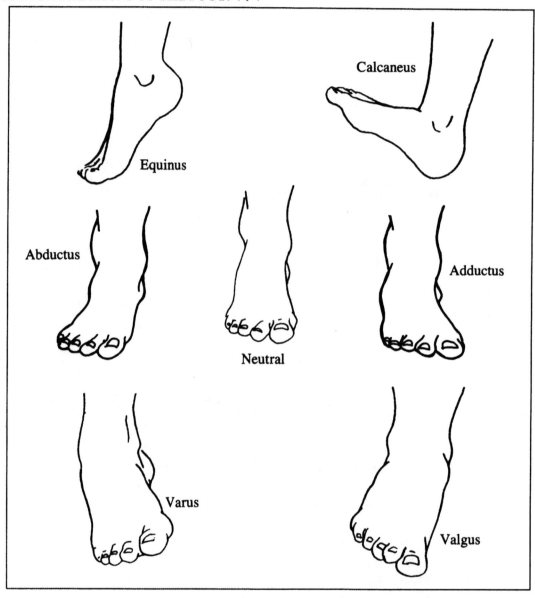

Calcaneus - a fixed position of dorsiflexion
Equinus - a fixed position of plantarflexion
Adductus - a fixed position of adduction
Abductus - a fixed position of abduction
Varus - a fixed position of inversion
Valgus - a fixed position of eversion

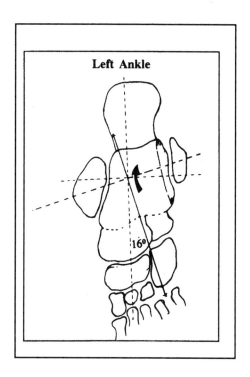

Left Ankle

16°

FUNCTION OF THE SUBTALAR AXIS

The subtalar axis is a 45 degree angle to the floor in the neutral position, about which the calcaneus rotates in relation to the talus and has a 16 degree angle medial to a line drawn through the second metatarsal.

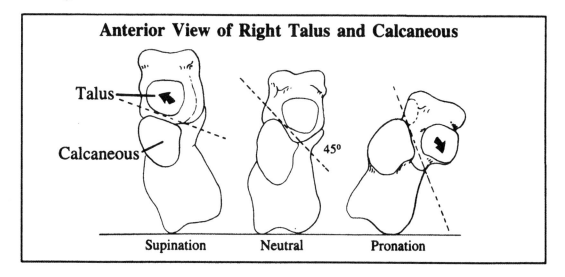

Anterior View of Right Talus and Calcaneous

Talus

Calcaneous

45°

Supination   Neutral   Pronation

Three types of movement occur about this subtalar axis:

1. Longitudinal axis = 8 to 12 degrees

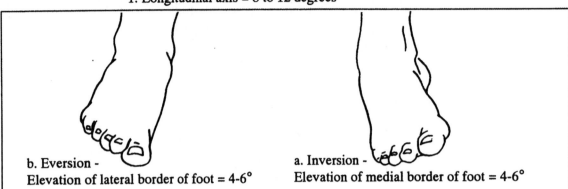

b. Eversion -
Elevation of lateral border of foot = 4-6°

a. Inversion -
Elevation of medial border of foot = 4-6°

2. Vertical axis

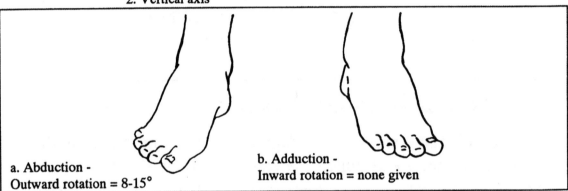

a. Abduction -
Outward rotation = 8-15°

b. Adduction -
Inward rotation = none given

3. Transverse axis - Much less than talus on tibia = 30 degrees

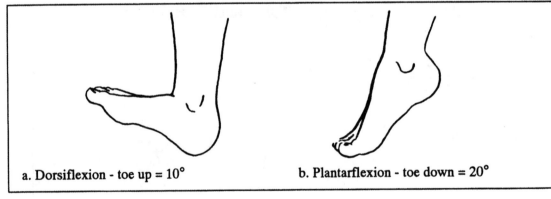

a. Dorsiflexion - toe up = 10°

b. Plantarflexion - toe down = 20°

Combinations of these three types of movement are:

1. Supination = Inversion, adduction, plantarflexion.

2. Pronation = Eversion, abduction, dorsiflexion.

CLOSED CHAIN MOTION OF THE SUBTALAR JOINT

PRONATION – 5 degrees

Calcaneus - Everts
Talus   - Adducts & plantar flexes
Leg   - Internally rotates & shortens
Knee   - Flexes & everts - valgus

(43, p. 4)

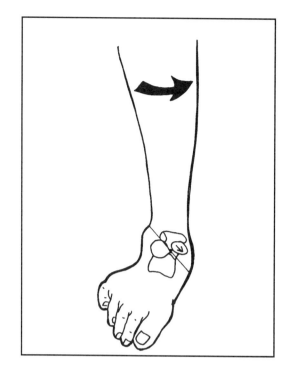

CLOSED CHAIN MOTION OF THE SUBTALAR JOINT

SUPINATION – 5 degrees

Calcaneus - Inverts
Talus   - Abducts & dorsiflexes
Leg   - Externally rotates &
              elongates
Knee   - Extends & inverts - varus

(43, p. 4)

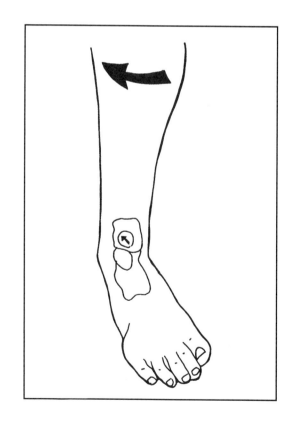

X-RAYS OF THE FOOT (58,p.57-59)

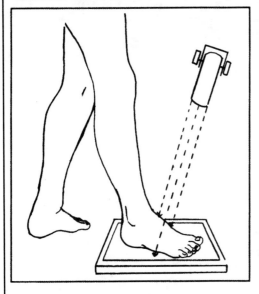

Dorsiplantar Foot Projection

Film Size   10 x 12 inches (24 x 30 cm)
Central Ray Through the base of the third metatarsal with ten degrees cephalad tube tilt.

Medial Oblique Foot Projection

Film Size   10 x 12 inches (24 x 30 cm)
Central Ray Through the base of the third metatarsal with no tube tilt.

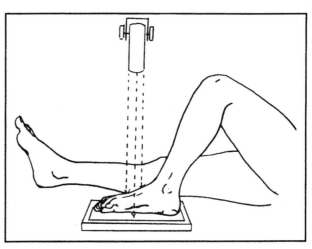

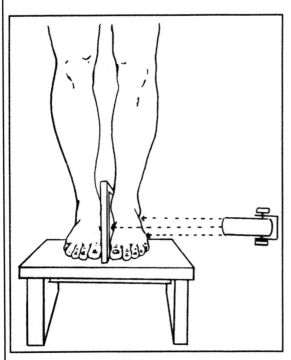

Lateral Foot Projection

Film Size   8 x 10 inches (18 x 24 cm) or larger if foot size requires it
Central Ray Through the medial navicular prominence.

REAR FOOT SUBLUXATIONS
CALCANEAL RANGE OF MOTION
IT IS AS SIMPLE AS ROCK AND ROLL

ROCK: While stabilizing the mid foot grasp the calcaneus and rock it into inversion and eversion. This checks the sub talar joint motion. Lack of inversion is adjusted into the lateral calcaneus. Lack of eversion is adjusted into the medial calcaneus at the sustentaculum tali.

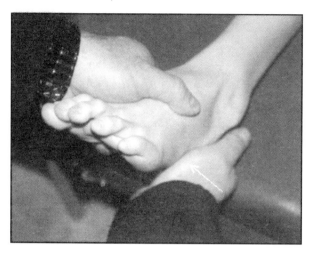 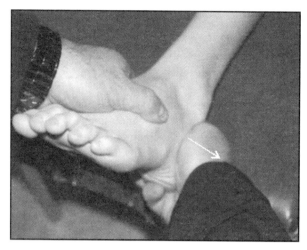

ROLL: Now adduct and abduct the calcaneus in relation to the cuboid using the same grip as above. Limitation in either direction results in a postero-lateral cuboid adjustment typically.

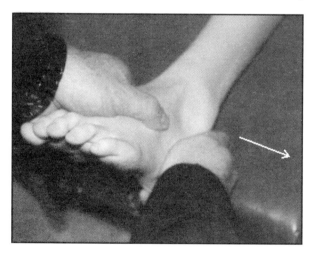 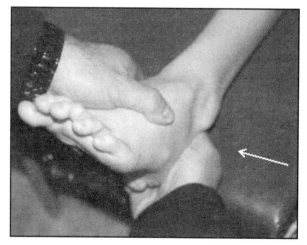

ADJUSTMENTS OF TALOCALCANEAL JOINT:

In neutral position, the calcaneus should be vertical and the sustentaculum tali should be horizontal.

SIGNS

1. Fixation upon motion palpation while side bending the calcaneus medially and laterally then internal and external rotation
2. Hypermobility
3. Pain at calcaneotibial or spring ligaments (medial)
4. Pain at calcaneofibular or calcaneocuboid ligaments (lateral)

DIFFERENTIAL DIAGNOSIS: *RULE THESE OUT*

. Ankle sprain
. Avulsion fracture

MEDIAL CALCANEUS:

SIGNS

Fixation or excess motion of calcaneus in relation to the talus, cuboid or spring ligament, with pain upon pressure at these joints or ligament.

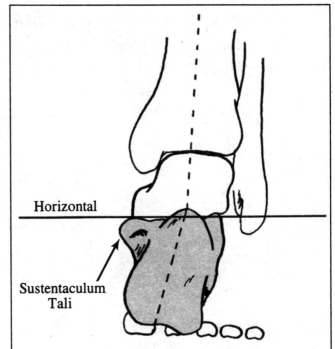

Rearfoot Varus due to non vertical calcaneus while horizontal plane of Sustentaculum Tali is present.

IMPACT OF INJURY

Weak heel counters of shoes fail to support the calcaneus. Chronic repetitive trauma of distance running or take off leg when jumping. Severe ankle sprains.

STABILIZATION

Face the bottom of the feet, and grasp the top of the forefoot with the hand to its lateral side. Place it against the inside of your flexed knee on the same side of your stabilization hand.

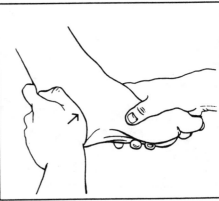

CONTACT & THRUST

With your thumb's metacarpo phalangeal prominence, contact the sustentaculum tali while your fingers grasp around the head of the calcaneus. Traction the foot and thrust at 90 degrees to the articulation directly laterally.

POST CHECKS

Normal motion should be restored if it was fixated with a 50% pain reduction in the previously tender adjacent joints.

LATERAL CALCANEUS:

SIGNS

Fixated or hypermobile with pain at the talocalcaneal joint and the calcaneal cuboid joint.

IMPACT OF INJURY

Hyperpronation and eversion ankle sprains.

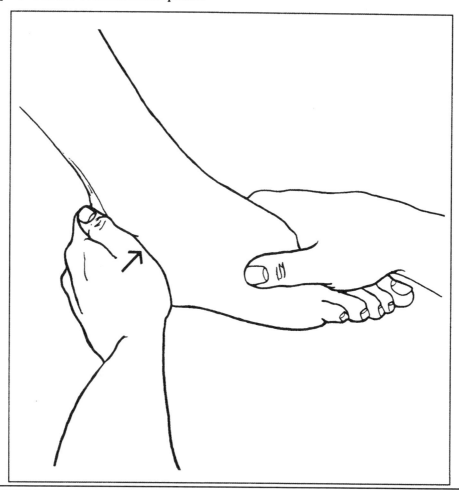

STABILIZATION

Face the bottom of the feet and grasp the top of the forefoot with the hand to its medial side. Now place it against the inside of the Dr.'s knee on that same side.

CONTACT & THRUST

With your thenar pad, contact the massive lateral surface of the calcaneus. With your fingers around the head of the calcaneus, traction and thrust medially.

POST CHECKS

Normal motion should be restored if there was a subluxation or fixation, pain should be 50% reduced in the previously tender adjacent joints.

THE MID FOOT

TRANSVERSE TARSAL JOINT/MIDTARSAL/CHOPART'S/"SURGEON'S TARSAL JOINT"
(5,p.10,11; 43,p.41-46; 56,p.459-471)

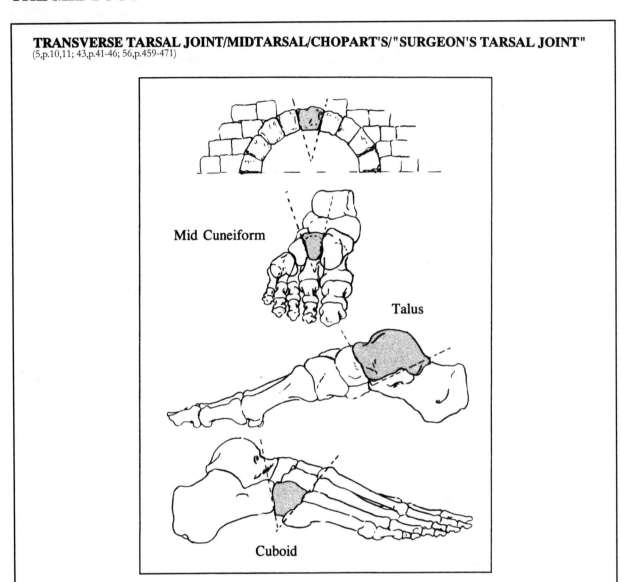

STRUCTURE OF THE MID FOOT

Five bones that transfer and adapt to forces from the rearfoot through locking mechanisms in their facets.

Talonavicular Joint: The convex head of the talus fits into the concave body of the navicular.

Navicularcuboid Joint: The lateral navicular is supported by the cuboid.

Calcanealcuboid Joint: This wedge shaped bone in front of the calcaneus has a proximal superior prominence that locks against the calcaneal facet as ground reaction forces push it up and drive it into the navicular bone.

Three cuneiforms: Extensions of the navicular longitudinally into the metatarsal bases, the transverse arch is supported laterally by the cuboid which lifts them when under load and assists the foot into abduction during gait.

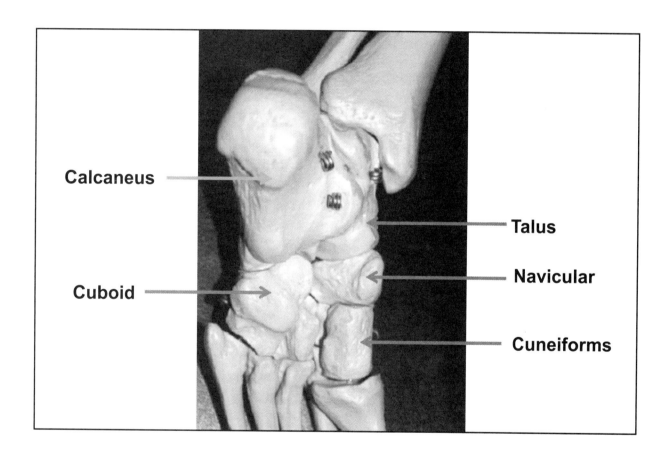

LIGAMENTS OF THE MIDFOOT - *NOT INCLUDING CAPSULAR LIGAMENTS*

1. Interosseous   - Holds together the transverse arch of the middle five tarsals.
2. Talonavicular   - Connects neck of talus to the dorsal surface of the navicular bone.
3. Calcaneocuboid   - A group that connects the dorsal and plantar surfaces of the calcaneus, cuboid, and metatarsals.
4. Calcaneonavicular   - (Spring Ligament) A bifurcated band that ties the calcaneus to the navicular bone.

FUNCTION OF THE MIDFOOT:

It allows accommodation to the uneven surfaces upon which man walks, and gives support while standing.

ADJUSTMENTS OF MID-TARSAL JOINTS:

The navicular and cuboid shapes determine the direction of traction when setting them up for the adjustment.

* *These adjustments are also what is used for the cuneiforms and the proximal metatarsal bases.*

SIGNS

- The bone involved is surrounded by painful joints
- Weakness of muscles inserting into subluxated mid tarsal bones
- Muscles will test strong if plastic deformation occurred
- A lump (if anterior)
- Indented (if posterior)
- Fixated upon shear stress
- Hypermobile upon shear stress

DIFFERENTIAL DIAGNOSIS

1. Tendon ruptures
2. Avulsion fractures
3. Congenital anomalies

MIDTARSAL ADJUSTMENTS

NAVICULAR ANTERIOR:

SIGNS

X-rays demonstrate a raise of 2mm or greater from the anterior talus head. Fixated or hypermobile with the talus and pain between the two bones to palpation. Weakness of the posterior tibial muscle.

IMPACT OF INJURY

Getting stepped on by human or animal. Kicking a hard object. Poor supporting shoes.

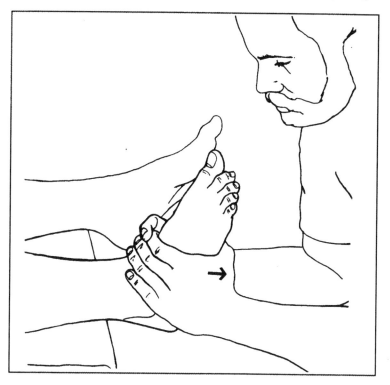

STABILIZATION

Grasping over fingers of contact hand on opposite side of foot.

CONTACT & THRUST

Place middle finger over the navicular, and your thumb on the ball of the foot. Press the foot down, so that the leg presses into the table before thrusting, then pull quickly inferior.

The purpose of pressing the leg into the table is to isolate the joint from yanking on the knee and hip as much as possible.

POST CHECKS

Restored motion if it was fixated, with reduction of palpatory pain at the talonavicular joint. A strong posterior tibial muscle.

75

NAVICULAR MEDIAL:

SIGNS

A more prominent medial and sore navicular bone. Weak posterior tibial muscle.

IMPACT OF INJURY

Excess foot pronation or forefoot abductus from medial to lateral foot trauma.

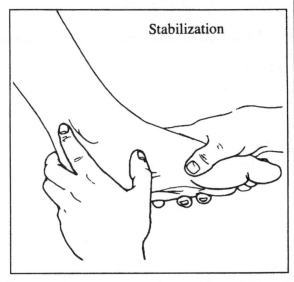

Stabilization

STABILIZATION

Grasping forefoot with lateral hand and tractioning inferiorly and laterally.

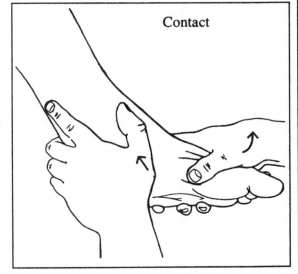

Contact

CONTACT & THRUST

With thenar eminence, contact the medial navicular with your fingers around the head of the calcaneus. Thrust superiorly so that your thumb slides up the anterior tibia while flexing the forefoot laterally.

POST CHECKS

A less prominent and better feeling medial navicular. Strong posterior tibial muscle.

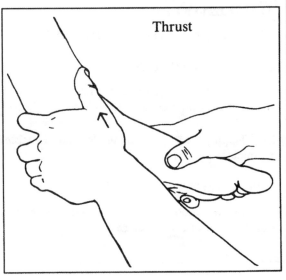

Thrust

NAVICULAR IS THE MOST PROMINENT BONE ON THE MEDIAL SIDE OF THE FOOT.

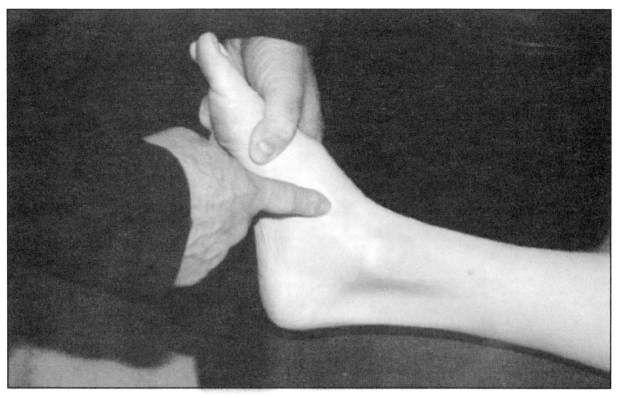

WITH THE THUMB METACARPAL PHALANGEAL JOINT ABOUT TO THRUST INTO THE NAVICULAR.

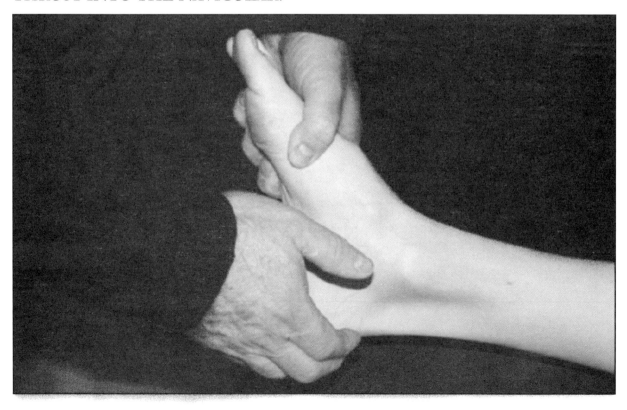

FOLLOW THROUGH WITH THE THRUST TO FREE THE FIXATION OF THE NAVICULAR.

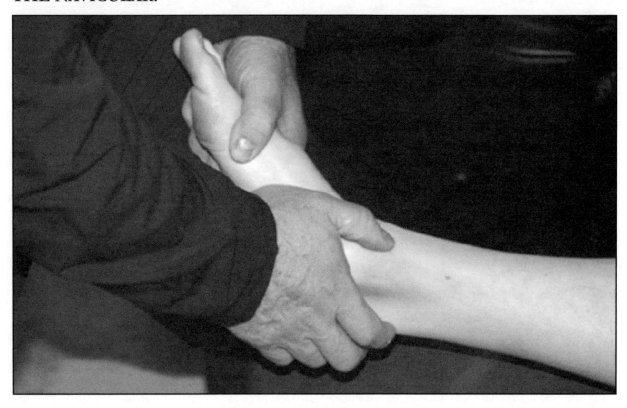

CONTACT & THRUST

With thenar eminence, contact the medial navicular with your fingers around the head of the calcaneus. Thrust superiorly so that your thumb slides up the anterior tibia while flexing the forefoot laterally.

POST CHECKS

A less prominent and better feeling medial navicular. Strong posterior tibial muscle.

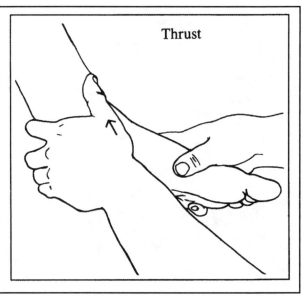

Thrust

CUBOID ANTERIOR:

SIGNS

Fixated or hypermobile cuboid with pain at its articular surfaces, creating a lump on top of the foot. Weak peroneus muscle.

IMPACT OF INJURY

Stepping on the sharp edge of a board or a rock.

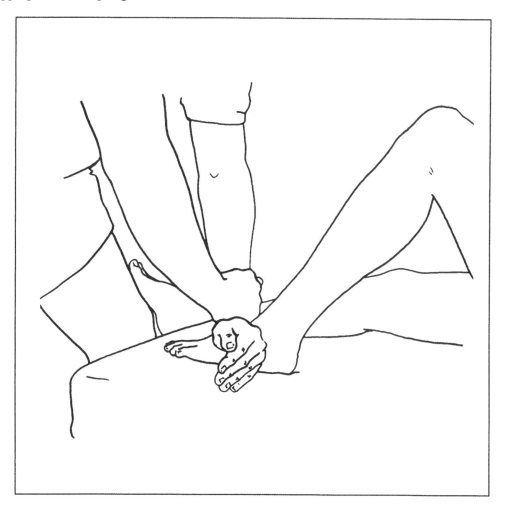

STABILIZATION

Grasping wrist of contact hand.

CONTACT & THRUST

A pisiform contact on top of the cuboid with a toggle recoil thrust.

POST CHECKS

Normal motion with a reduced lump and pain. Strong peroneus muscle.

CUBOID LOCATED JUST PROXIMAL TO THE FIFTH METATARSAL STYLOID PROCESS.

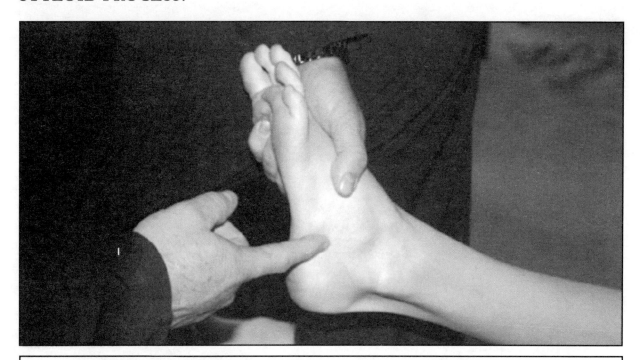

CUBOID POSTERO-LATERAL

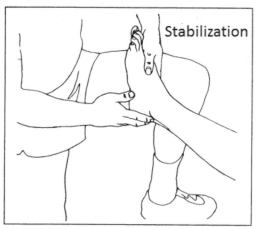

Stabilization

This adjustment is easier to perform if you utilize the wedge shape of the cuboid and flex the rearfoot and forefoot laterally toward the cuboid.

SIGNS

Painful adjacent joints with no obvious lump or indentation. Weak peroneus muscle.

IMPACT OF INJURY

Forefoot stepped on from lateral side. Side kick in karate.

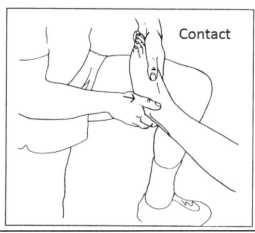

Contact

STABILIZATION

Grasping forefoot with medial hand and tractioning.

CUBOID LATERAL:

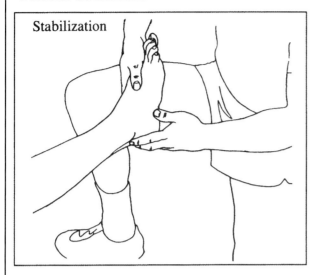

Stabilization

This adjustment is easier to perform if you utilize the wedge shape of the cuboid and flex the rearfoot and forefoot laterally toward the cuboid.

SIGNS

Painful adjacent joints with no obvious lump or indentation. Weak peroneus muscle.

IMPACT OF INJURY

Forefoot stepped on from lateral side. Side kick in karate.

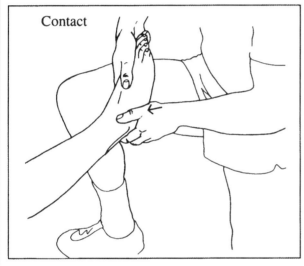

Contact

STABILIZATION

Grasping forefoot with medial hand and tractioning.

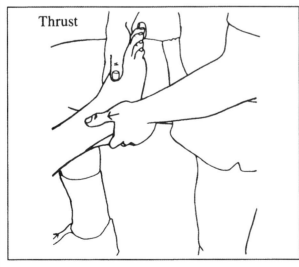

Thrust

CONTACT & THRUST

With your thenar eminence contact the lateral cuboid with your fingers around the calcaneus. Thrust superiorly so that your thumb glides along the anterior fibula while flexing the forefoot laterally.

POST CHECKS

Reduced pain of adjacent joint spaces with normal motion. Strong peroneus muscle.

THE THUMB METACARPAL PHALANGEAL JOINT IS USED TO THRUST INTO THE CUBOID.

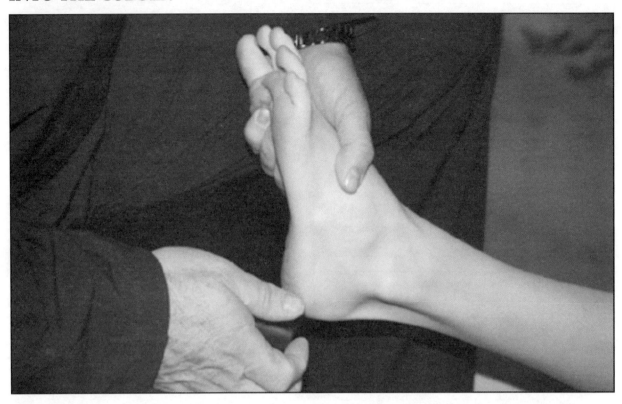

THE THRUST FOLLOWS THROUGH INTO THE CUBOID TO FREE THE FIXATION

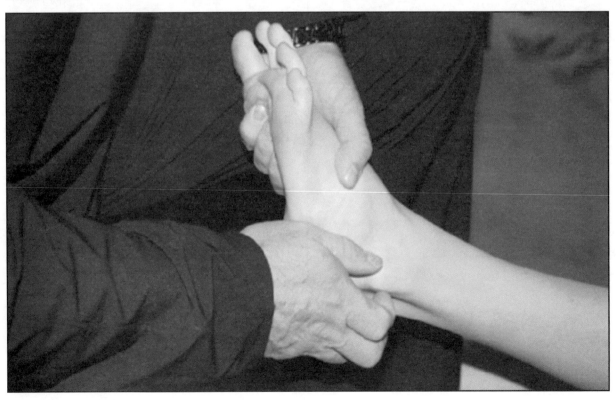

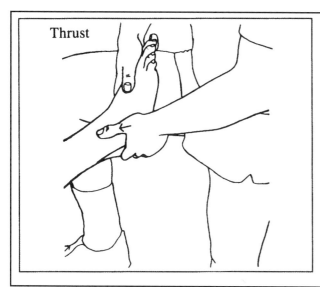

Thrust

CONTACT & THRUST

With your thenar eminence contact the lateral cuboid with your fingers around the calcaneus. Thrust superiorly so that your thumb glides along the anterior fibula while flexing the forefoot laterally.

POST CHECKS

Reduced pain of adjacent joint spaces with normal motion. Strong peroneus muscle.

POSTERIOR TARSAL

This is by far the most frequent midfoot subluxation. During walking the forces into your foot are 1 to 3 times your body weight. During running, the forces are from 3 to 5 times your body weight. During vertical leap sports such as volleyball or basketball the forces can reach levels of 5 to 7 times your body weight.

Now what are the chances of you getting your feet stepped on in athletic competition? What kind of force is going into your foot when it is stepped on? Do you think that maybe someone should know how to correct foot subluxations that are being created by these forces?

Learning the following adjustment will be a big step toward helping these people.

POSTERIOR MIDTARSALS AND METATARSAL BASES:

SIGNS

On X-ray, a 2mm or greater drop from the more proximal segment. A palpable stair stepping down from the proximal segment with pain at that joint to palpation. Fixation or hypermobility on shear stress motion. A weak posterior tibial muscle.

IMPACT OF INJURY

Getting stepped on by man or beast. Kicking hard objects. Poor tarsal arch support in shoe.

POSTERIOR TARSAL LANDMARKS

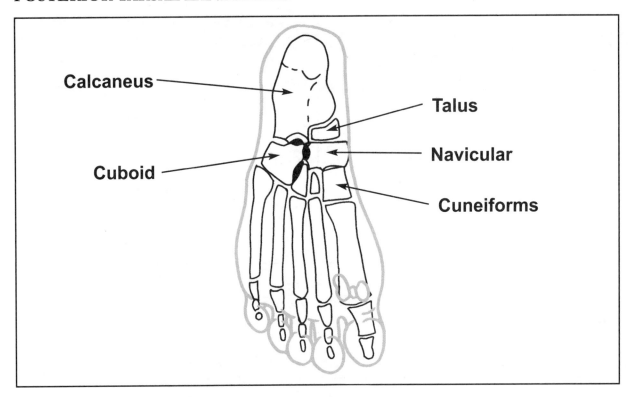

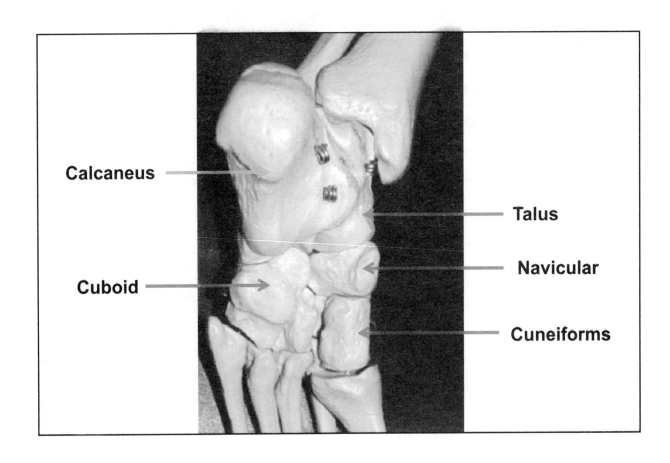

STABILIZATION

With the patient prone, you grasp the opposite side of the forefoot from the contact hand and place your thumb or pisiform directly over the contact thumb.

CONTACT & THRUST

Place your thumb on the sole of the foot under the bone that is posterior. Grasp the forefoot with your fingers then add the stabilization hand. Traction the foot down into the table so that the forefoot is being pulled away from the hind foot, then thrust anteriorly with your thumbs and or pisiform.

POST CHECKS

A more even joint alignment with better motion and less pain. A strong posterior tibial muscle.

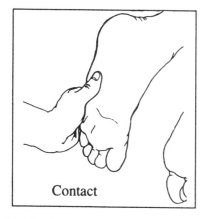
Contact

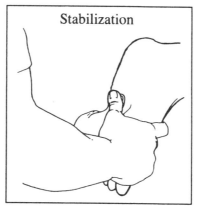
Stabilization

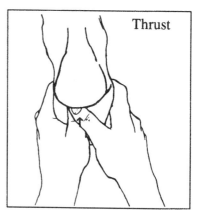
Thrust

OVERCOMING THE REPUTATION

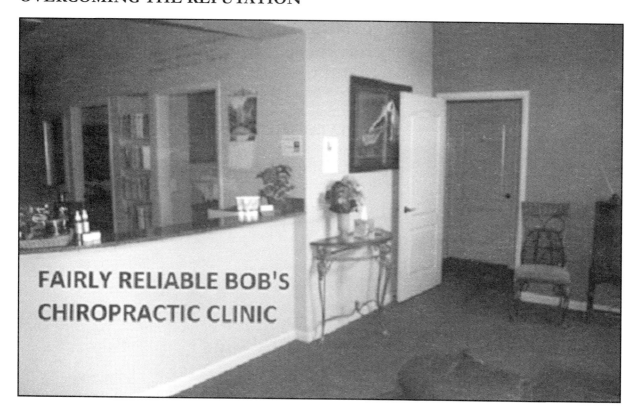

FAIRLY RELIABLE BOB'S CHIROPRACTIC CLINIC

FOREFOOT / ANTERIOR FOOT 19 BONES
14 PHALANGES AND 5 METATARSALS

Note the proximal end of the metatarsals help make up the transverse arch however the metatarsal heads themselves may be flat against the ground or shoe.

(5,p.12-15; 4,p,46-54; 41,p. 461-471)

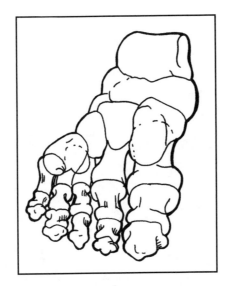

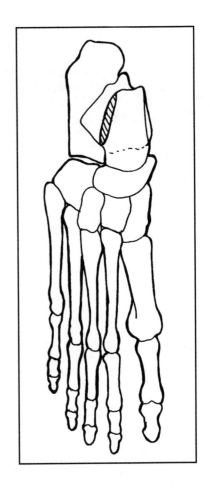

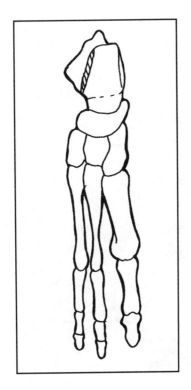

MEDIAL FOREFOOT

1ST METATARSAL: The thickest and shortest metatarsal, but third in length in terms of forward projection. The proximal base is kidney shaped allowing dorsi and plantar flexion including rotation about an arc around the base of the second metatarsal.

2nd METATARSAL: The longest metatarsal that protrudes the farthest. Because of its length it bears weight readily.

3rd METATARSAL: The second longest metatarsal in forward projection.

(5,p.12-15; 4,p,46-54; 41,p. 461-471)

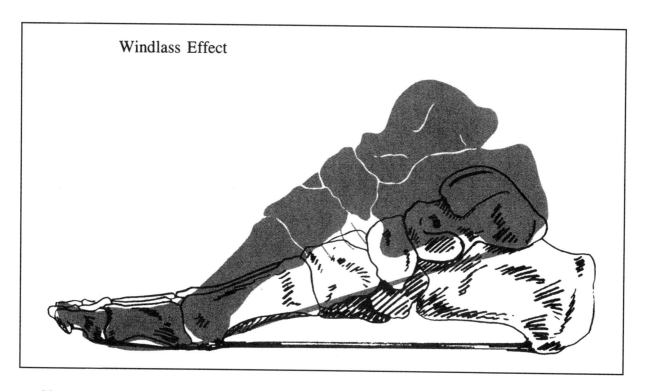

Windlass Effect

Two accessory bones act as a fulcrum on the plantar surface of the 1st met head for the tendons of the flexor halluces brevis and plantar fascia and they bear body weight. It is the fulcrum that allows the windlass effect to supinate the foot.

Attaching to the plantar surface are the anterior tibia and peroneus longus tendons into the 1st cuneiform.

(5,p.12-15; 4,p,46-54; 41,p. 461-471)

LATERAL FOREFOOT

4th Metatarsal: The fourth longest metatarsal in projection.

5th Metatarsal: The shortest in projection but ample motion about a tri plane axis in directions of supination and pronation and probably is third in weight bearing.

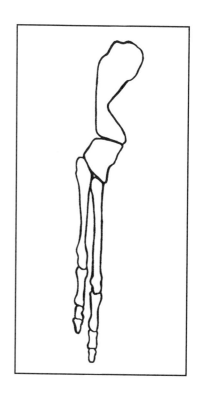

FUNCTION OF THE METATARSALS:

They allow gliding of articular surfaces through pronation and supination, locking the tarsals when they are in full pronation and assisting the supination process as a fulcrum for the plantar fascia.

You just read a very profound statement that I am afraid you may pass by too quickly, without some contemplation about how it relates to the illustrations on this page.

Consider the fulcrum at the ball of the foot and how the toes would draw tight the plantar fascia as they dorsiflex in relation to the metatarsal heads. This would shorten the foot's length by drawing the heel toward the metatarsal heads.

Imagine how this motion would change due to fixation or hypermobility of the metatarsal shafts at either end.

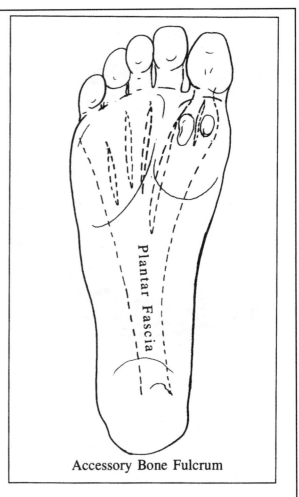

Plantar Fascia

Accessory Bone Fulcrum

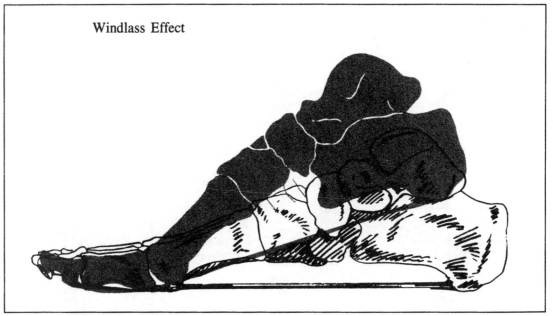

Windlass Effect

The arch can only raise if the joints can glide and respond to the tightening of the plantar fascia during heel raise.

88

WINDLASS EFFECT BLOCKED

If the mid foot joints don't glide, then the fascia jams the toes into the met heads, effectively blocking the windlass, and leads to hammer or claw toes. It may also pull the big toe lateral and develop a bunion. These are just a few of the problems a blocked windlass develops.

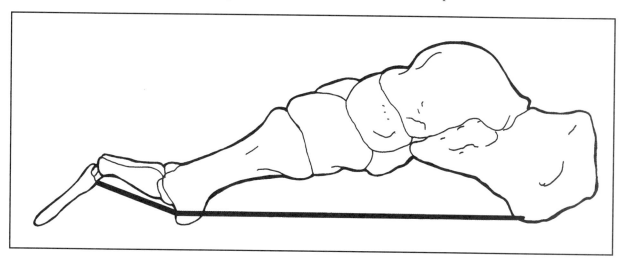

FUNCTIONAL HALLUX LIMITUS (F.H.L.) .(6, p.650; 7, p.12-14; 8, p.54)

The normal big toe can dorsiflex, when not under load, from 70 to 90 degrees. When it is loaded with weight in the pronated position, this can drastically change with many individuals. The big toe may lock at 20 degrees of dorsiflexion effectively blocking normal supination and the windlass effect. If the first ray is allowed to plantar flex at

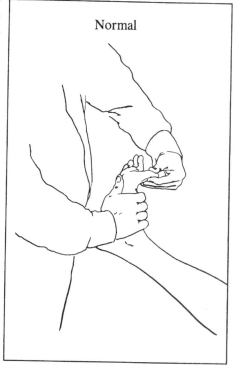

Normal

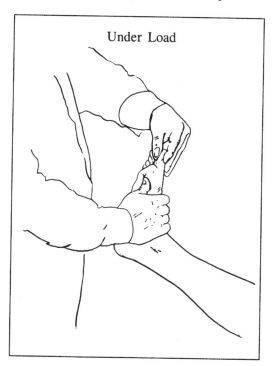

Under Load

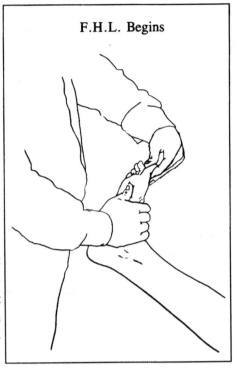

F.H.L. Begins

this point, it usually allows further dorsiflexion of the big toe and enhances supination and the windlass effect. But due to the design of most shoes and foot orthotics, this does not happen. Therefore, __functional hallux limitus can be defined as the functional inability of the proximal phalanx of the hallux to extend on the first metatarsal head when under load.__

To test this place your thumb under the first ray just proximal to the sesamoid bones. Press the first ray into dorsiflexion. Now dorsiflex the big toe and observe at what angle it begins to force your thumb down, that is under the first ray. This is the moment that F.H.L. begins.

ADJUSTMENTS OF FOREFOOT:

The metatarsals and phalanges get a lot of forces that can rotate them as well as subluxate them anterior or posterior, such as getting stepped on, or kicking something, or simply stepping on a rock. Because the adjustments for anterior and posterior are the same as the previous tarsals, I will only describe the rotational maneuvers for the proximal metatarsals. The distal metatarsals and phalanges will be given their normal description.

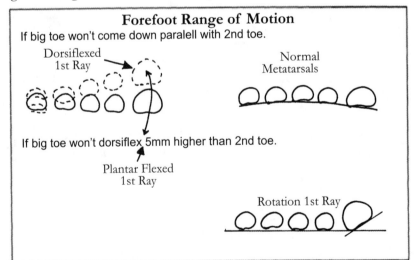

Forefoot Range of Motion
If big toe won't come down paralell with 2nd toe.

Dorsiflexed 1st Ray

Normal Metatarsals

If big toe won't dorsiflex 5mm higher than 2nd toe.

Plantar Flexed 1st Ray

Rotation 1st Ray

Dorsiflexed and plantarflexed 1st rays are usually a result of the fixated tarsal arch structure.

DORSIFLEXED AND PLANTARFLEXED 1ST RAY

It is normal for the first ray (met head) to come down parallel to the second met head. If it can't it is considered **a dorsiflexed first ray.**

It is also normal for the first ray to dorsiflex at least 5mm higher than the second ray. If it can't it is considered **a plantarflexed first ray.**

I am of the opinion that most of these conditions are simply a result of fixated bones in the midfoot and respond well to adjustments of the feet.

(22) [Glasoe WM, Yack HJ, Saltzman CL. Anatomy and biomechanics of the first ray. Phys Ther. 1999;79:854–859.]

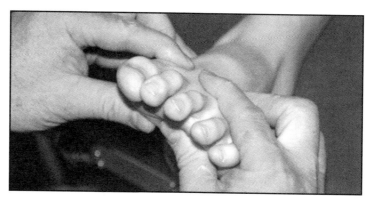

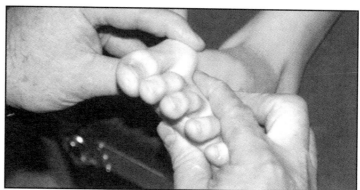

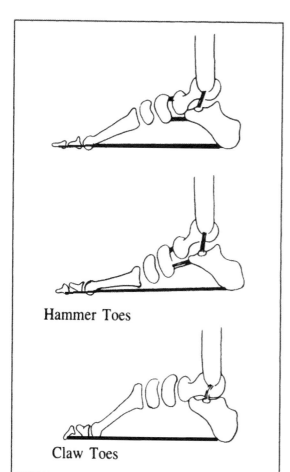

Hammer Toes

Claw Toes

SIGNS OF METATARSAL SUBLUXATION:

1. Pain at metatarsal base
2. Toe nail turned medial or lateral
3. Hallux valgus
4. Thick yellow toe nail from lack of trophic supply
5. Pinch callus
6. Flat metatarsal arch
7. Mallet toes, Hammer toes or Claw toes
8. Less than **5** mm dorsiflexion of the 1st ray M.T.P. relative to the 2nd ray M.T.P. joint
9. Inability of the 1st ray M.T.P. to plantar flex so it is even with the 2nd ray M.T.P. joint

DIFFERENTIAL DIAGNOSIS: *RULE THESE OUT*

1. Hallux limitus
2. Bunion
3. Forefoot valgus or varus
4. Wart
5. Morton's neuroma
6. Functional hallux limitus
7. Plantar flexed 1st ray
8. Dorsiflexed 1st ray

METATARSAL ROTATION

Look for a turned toe nail that also has tenderness to palpation in the interosseous space along the metatarsal shaft especially near the base.

The impact of injury is typically from being stepped on, especially with cleats, with momentum in the transverse plane. Please do not consider the little toe unless known trauma is significant at that site.

LOOK FOR TOENAIL ROTATION

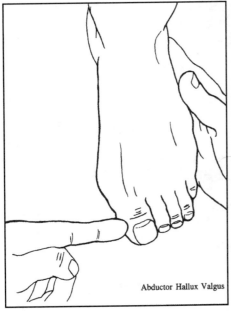

Abductor Hallux Valgus

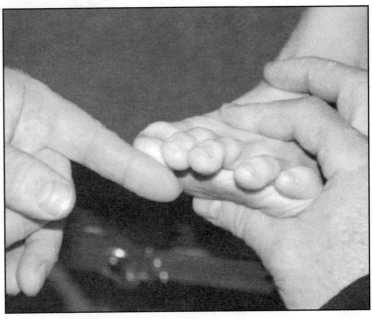

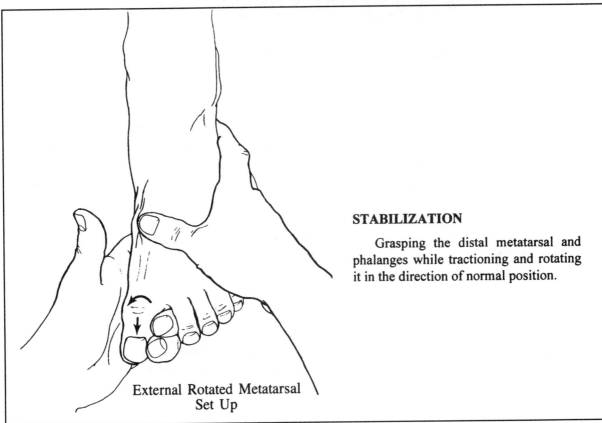

External Rotated Metatarsal
Set Up

STABILIZATION

Grasping the distal metatarsal and phalanges while tractioning and rotating it in the direction of normal position.

CONTACT & THRUST

Place your thumb on the proximal metatarsal base so that it pushes into the same side that the toe nail has turned toward. This will cause it to de-rotate. The fingers of this hand may squeeze the bottom of the foot to increase thumb pressure.

POST CHECKS

Toe nail is level with the other toe nails now and interossei muscles feel much less painful along with the joint.

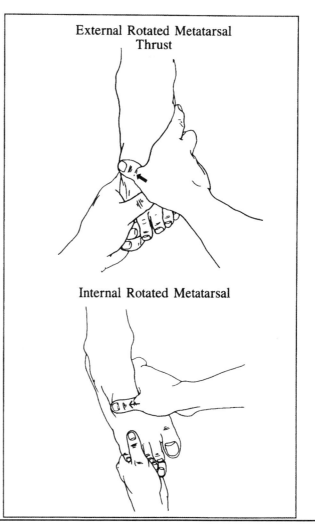

External Rotated Metatarsal Thrust

Internal Rotated Metatarsal

PROXIMAL PHALANX / METATARSAL HEAD SUBLUXATION

This adjustment is identical to the orthopedic test called Strunsky's Sign. If lancinating pain occurs while performing this at the metatarsal phalangeal joints, it is indicative of metatarsalgia. It is both diagnostic as well as therapeutic.

Signs include sore metatarsal heads with calluses under the middle ones and often hammer toes.

Impact of injury includes poor shock absorbing shoes and also poor dorsiflexion of the big toe when under load. Tightening of the plantar fascia due to locked midfoot joints compresses the toes against the metatarsal heads.

Only the 2nd through 5th met heads are adjusted and contacted.

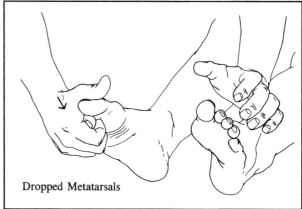

Dropped Metatarsals

CONTACT & THRUST

The base of the palm contacts the proximal dorsal 2-5 toes, while the fingers surround the distal toes and stabilizes against the ball of the foot. The thrust is given with a sudden palmar flexion of the wrist. Singularly this can be done by isolating one toe with the thumb and finger.

POST CHECK

Following a series of at least five adjustments over a two week period or more, Strunsky's Sign should be negative or much reduced. Toe flexibility should increase.

If it is painful the first time you perform this adjustment, I have found that by the fifth adjustment the majority of patients do not mind having it done. In fact, most people say that walking is much easier afterward and they like how their feet are now feeling.

EXERCISES FOR THE TOES HELPS KEEP CONTROL OF FUNCTION AS WELL AS POSITION OF THE TOES.

TOE ADDUCTION	TOE ABDUCTION

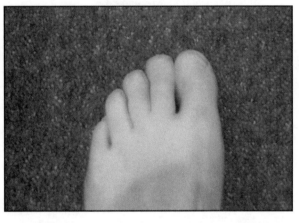 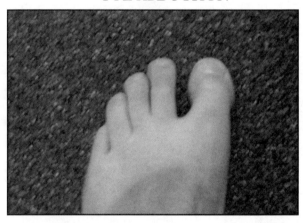

TOE ABDUCTION MAY BE ACTIVATED BY PULLING THE BIG TOE INTO ABDUCTION AND MASSAGING THE ABDUCTOR POLLICIS MUSCLE

STRENGTHENING THE ABDUCTOR POLLICIS CAN BE ACCOMPLISHED WITH RUBBER BAND EXERCISES

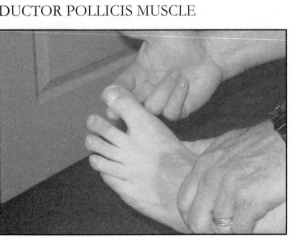 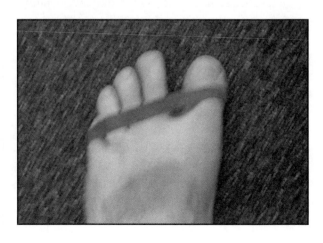

PHALANGES:

SIGNS

Fixation or hypermobility of the toes. Claw or hammer toes. Pain in the toe.

IMPACT OF INJURY

Getting stepped on, or short shoes that may be pointed.

STABILIZATION

Grasp the proximal bone of the joint being adjusted.

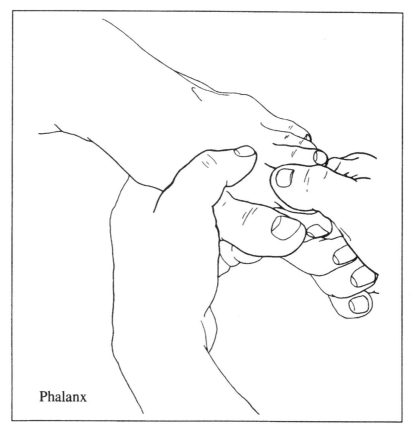

Phalanx

CONTACT & THRUST

While moving the distal phalanx through a circular motion, a fixation will be felt. At this time a gentle thrust is made into the fixation.

POST CHECK

Normal motion and reduced pain.

Remember that *energy goes where energy flows*, and callouses and bunions are an example of energy flowing and rubbing at these sites. Also remember that *energy stops where energy flops*, and baby soft skin where you would expect pressure to be applied is a sign of non-weight bearing.

STRETCHING OF THE PHALLANGES INTO EXTENTION CAN GIVE MORE FLEXI-
BILITY AND HELP PREVENT HAMMER TOES. MYOFASCIAL RELEASES ON THE SOLE
OF THE FOOT ARE ALSO QUITE HELPFUL.

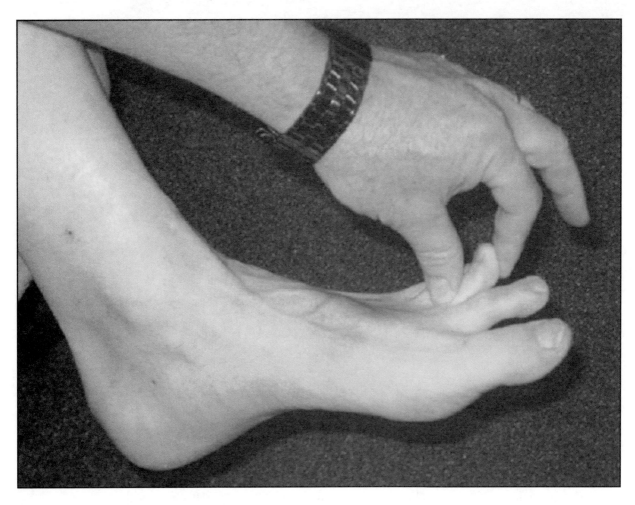

CHAPTER THIRTEEN

FOOT AND ANKLE RANGE OF MOTION (29, p.223-225)

    A. Ankle plantar flexion - 50 degrees
    B. Ankle dorsi flexion - 20 degrees
    C. Forefoot adduction / internal rotation - 20 degrees
    D. Forefoot abduction / external rotation - 10 degrees
    E. Subtalar inversion - 5 degrees
    F. Subtalar eversion - 5 degrees

FIRST METATARSOPHALANGEAL JOINT (8,p.226)

    A. Flexion - 45 degrees
    B. Extension - 70 to 90 degrees

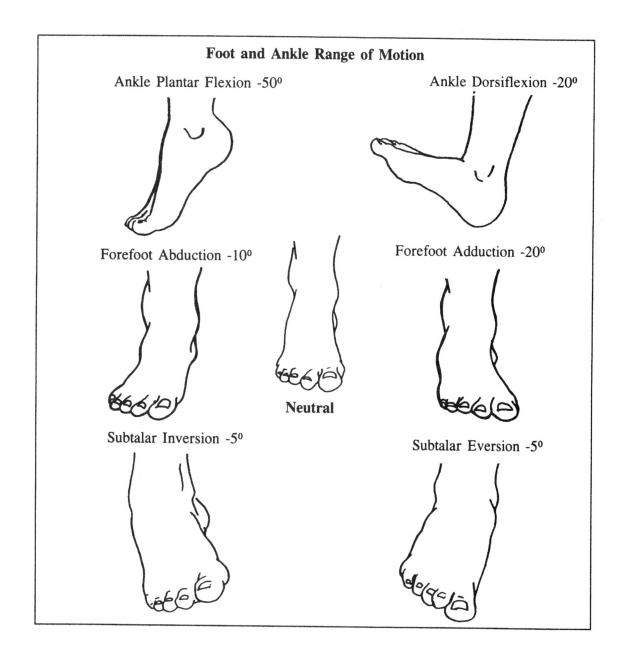

Foot and Ankle Range of Motion

Ankle Plantar Flexion -50°

Ankle Dorsiflexion -20°

Forefoot Abduction -10°

Neutral

Forefoot Adduction -20°

Subtalar Inversion -5°

Subtalar Eversion -5°

KEITH RAU (CENTER) & NANCY NORTH (RIGHT) WITH ME AT NCAA TRACK CHAMPIONSHIP.

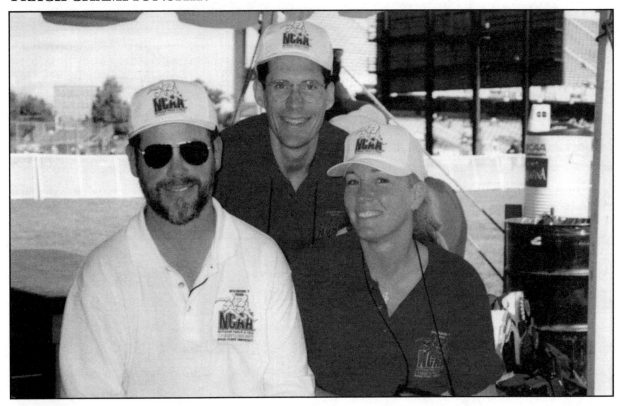

MY GAIT LAB

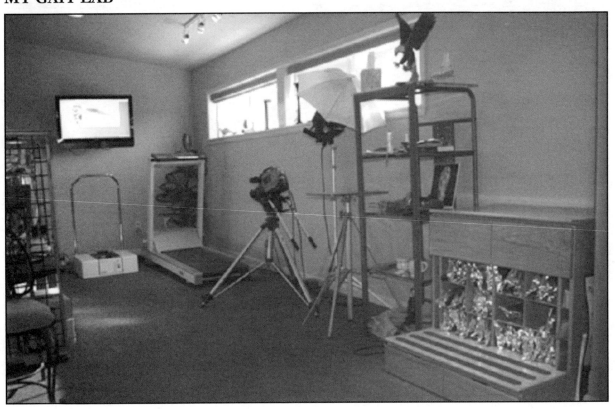

IMMEDIATE FEEDBACK WITH VIDEO IN REAL TIME

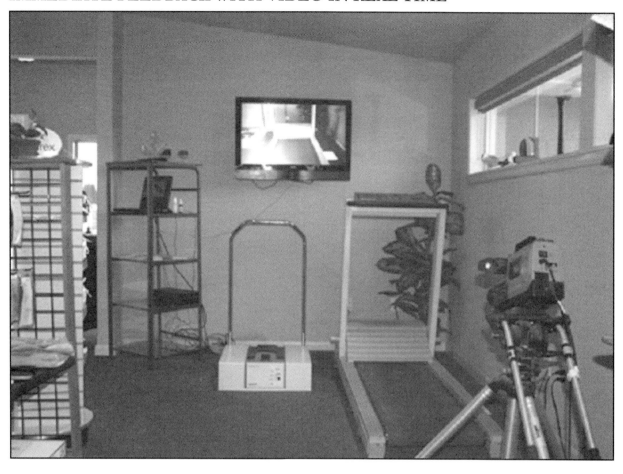

CHAPTER FOURTEEN
DEFINITIONS

SUBLUXATION: A partial dislocation produced by any motion in a joint that is contrary to its plane of motion, or that exceeds the range of motion of that joint while affecting its neuromuscular response. This position puts the ligament and capsule under stretch until plastic deformation occurs.

COMPENSATION: An abnormal change of structural position of one part in an attempt by the body to adjust to deviation of structure, position or function of another part.

HYPERMOBILITY: Instability and excessive motion at a joint, which should be stable when normal loads are applied.

FIXATION: Limited and restricted motion at a joint, which should be mobile when normal loads are applied.

HALLUX ABDUCTO-VALGUS

- Subluxation of the first metatarsal-phalangeal joint (MTP) in the transverse plane, secondary to dorsiflexion and inversion of the first ray.
- The pre-disposing factors are an adducted foot and abnormal pronation.
- Functional Hallux Limitus is frequently a predisposing factor when the big toe will not dorsiflex well under load.

ABDUCTO HALLUX VALGUS

Deviation of the hallux (big toe) at the Metacarpal Phalangeal joint laterally.

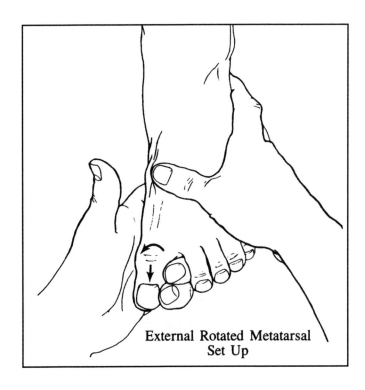

**External Rotated Metatarsal
Set Up**

HALLUX LIMITUS

Subluxation of the 1st metatarsal phalangeal joint (MTP) in the sagital plane, secondary to dorsiflexion of the 1st ray. This often result from a rectus foot and abnormal pronation, especially when it's a long 1st metacarpal. Hypermobility of the proximal phallanx is classic.

A rocker bottom shoe is a good choice for someone with this condition or if the big toe gets irritated easily

HALLUX RIGIDUS

The latter stage of hallux limitus, resulting in osteoarthritic joint changes leading to ankylosis of the 1st MTP joint.

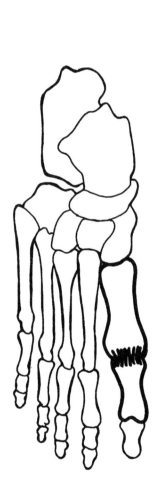

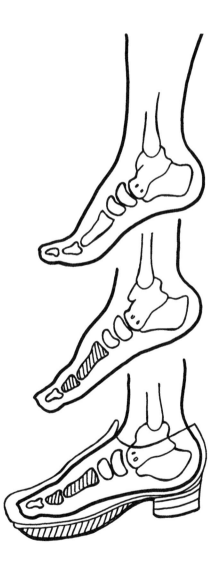

DEFINITIONS

Neuroma: A fibrosis of the neurovascular bundle due to shearing forces between the metatarsal heads and the plantar tissues. Most frequently occurs between the 3rd and 4th metatarsal heads.

Plantar Fascitis: Inflammation of the plantar fascia, usually at the calcaneus bone interface and spreading into the mid foot, due to excess tension from elongation of the foot when the medial tarsal arch drops and remains fixated stopping normal supination. Tearing of fascia fibers results as the heel raises on the toes fulcrum and no mid foot glide occurs superiorly suddenly jerking on the fascia.

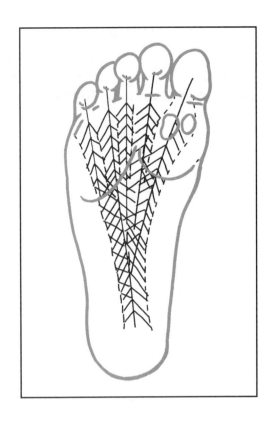

DR. MICHAEL PETTY U. OF TENNESSEE TEAM DR. AT NCAA TRACK & FIELD NAT. CHAMP

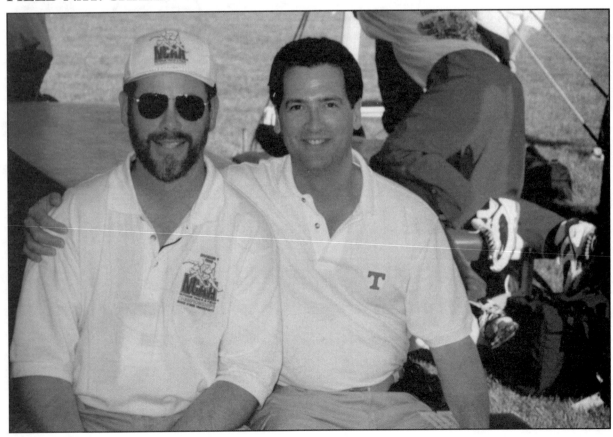

EXTRINSIC DEFORMITIES

- ROTATIONAL: Internal or external rotation of the bones of the lower extremity known as Tibial torsion or Femoral torsion. Rotations at the hip or knee joints. This is a transverse plane deformity.
- LEG LENGTH Discrepancies: Two Types; <u>Anatomic</u>- Structural shortage of the femur, tibia or foot, and sometimes all.

     <u>Physiologic</u>- A functional shortage due to structural mal-position or faulty posture of the back, pelvis, knee, ankle or foot.

TIBIA VARUM

- The distal tibia is deviated or bowed inward toward the midline of the body.
- A frontal plane deformity that pronates the subtalar joint.
- Frequently seen in "Bow Legs".

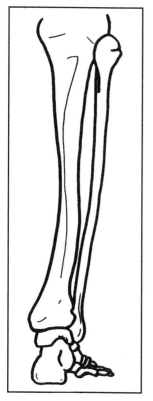

TIBIA VALGUM

- The distal tibia is deviated or bowed away from the midline of the body.
- A frontal plane deformity that supinates the subtalar joint.
- Frequently seen in "knock knees"..

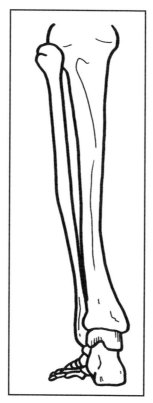

RECTUS OR STRAIGHT TIBIA

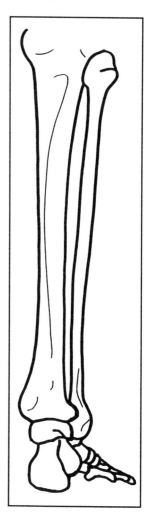

CHAPTER FIFTEEN

COMMON LOCATIONS OF PAIN

- Trochanteric Bursitis- Pain directly over the greater trochanter of the femur.
- T.F.L./Iliotibial Band Syndrome- Pain isolated to the lateral thigh.
- Bakers Cyst- Non-pulsating spongy mass behind the knee.
- Chondro Malacia Patella- Patella tracking pains (usually from vastus muscle imbalance or excessive pronation.) (30, p. 488-450; 33, p. 696-657)
- SHIN SPLINTS: Pain at musculo-tendonous junction of (either) the anterior (or posterior) leg. (Each compartment results from a different etiology.)
- COMPARTMENT SYNDROME: Pain which can be eliminated or made tolerable by exercise is not due to a compartment syndrome.
- Medial Tibial – Tender trigger points at medial border of the posterior tibia muscle during running, that disappear at rest.
- (Anterior Tibial – A painful tight sensation on the antero-lateral aspect of the leg in the peroneal group and anterior tibia muscle, with weakness of dorsiflexion.)
- SEVERS DISEASE: Calcaneal epiphysitis. Pain at the back of the heel in the mid teen years.
- ACHILLES TENDON: From over use or direct trauma or rupture. Be mindful of specific pain that may lead to focal degeneration and secondary thickening of the paratenon.
- Since the gastrocnemius attaches above the knee, it is functional with the leg extended and releases when the leg is flexed.
- The soleus origin attaches below the knee, and therefore is functional with the leg flexed.
- Plantar flexion of the foot in either leg position will help diagnose an injury to the proper portion of the tendon or muscle.
- ANKLE SPRAIN: Inversion is the most common. This is discussed well in the ankle ligament section.

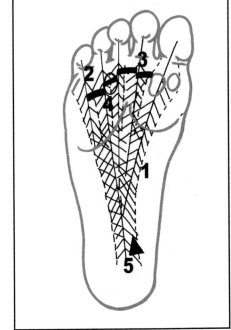

1. Plantar Fascitis – From flattening of the longitudinal tarsal arch.
2. Intertransverse Ligament Sprain – Secondary to #1.
3. Bursitis Between Metatarsal Heads – Secondary to #2.
4. Morton's Neuroma – Secondary to # 1,2,3.
5. Calcaneal Heel Spur – Secondary to # 1.

- STRESS FRACTURES: When uncontrolled pronation occurs during the gait cycle, shock absorption is no longer attenuated by normal pronation and knee flexion. Therefore greater shock is transmitted into the bone structure creating small painful breaks in the cortex and periosteum of the extremity. (KGH)

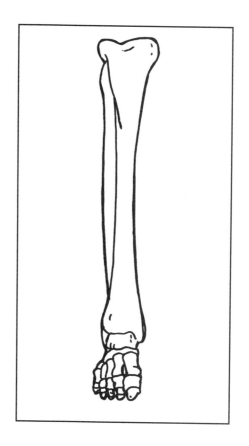

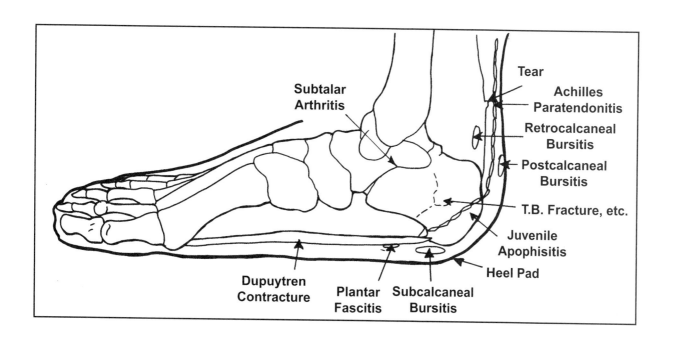

105

CHAPTER SIXTEEN

SHOE DEFINITIONS
GARY D. THOMPSON, C.P.O.

- HEEL COUNTER: The component of the shoe that is a molded unit that gives support to the back portion of the shoe around the heel.
- LAST: A mold or model over which a shoe is made ("shoe last"). Once the sole is made to this shape it's a "sole last". There are different styles of lasts for various shapes of feet.
- TOE BOX: The area in the front of the shoes that surrounds the toes.
- INSOLE: A liner placed inside a shoe for shock absorption and foot comfort. It is removable to allow for other materials or orthotics.

- ROCKER BOTTOM SOLE: Applied to the bottom of the sole to help rock the foot from heel strike to toe off without bending the shoe. This provides relief for metatarsal heads and hallusis rigidus (and functional hallux limitus).

- METATARSAL BAR: A material placed on the bottom of the sole which is designed to decrease pressure on the metatarsal heads. (This decreases dorsiflexion of the toes and therefore decreases plantar fascia tightening.) The first and fifth metatarsal heads are used as landmarks to position various types of metatarsal bars.

- EXTRA DEPTH SHOE: A shoe that is deeper by ¼" to ¾". This allows extra room for special insoles or orthotics.

- THOMAS HEEL: A heel that typically has an anterior medial extension of ½" longer than the standard heel. It's purpose is to give added leverage for support under the susentaculum tali. A medial wedge (post) may also be used if additional support is necessary. (Application: Infants or children with outtoeing {duck feet} or forefoot valgus.)The Thomas Heel can also be used laterally (hence reversed Thomas Heel) to give support to the cuboid area. This will tend to externally rotate the foot. (Application: Infants or children with intoeing {pigeon toes}or forefoot varus.)

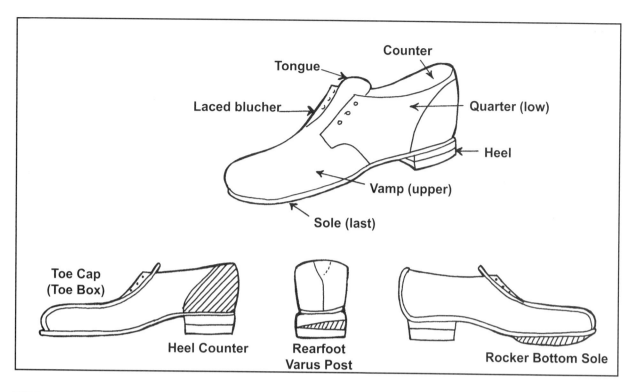

Counter

Tongue

Laced blucher

Quarter (low)

Heel

Vamp (upper)

Sole (last)

Toe Cap
(Toe Box)

Heel Counter

Rearfoot
Varus Post

Rocker Bottom Sole

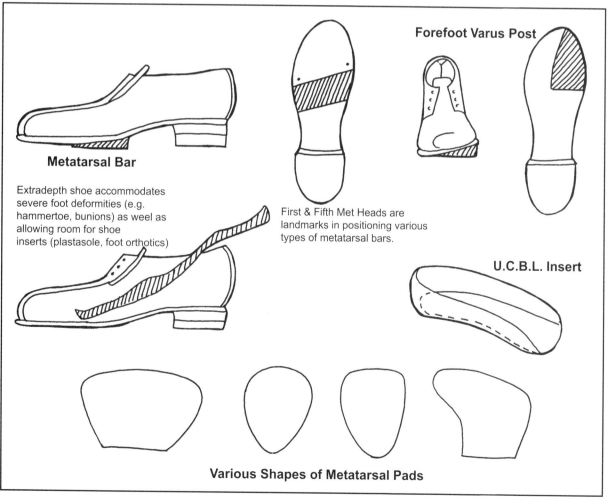

Forefoot Varus Post

Metatarsal Bar

Extradepth shoe accommodates
severe foot deformities (e.g.
hammertoe, bunions) as weel as
allowing room for shoe
inserts (plastasole, foot orthotics)

First & Fifth Met Heads are
landmarks in positioning various
types of metatarsal bars.

U.C.B.L. Insert

Various Shapes of Metatarsal Pads

A GOOD SHOE

- Should flex where the foot flexes, at the ball of the foot. It should not flex into the arch area.
- Do not assume that the other shoe will pass after examining one shoe.
- The heel counter should have a strength level of at least 5 on a 10 point scale.

PICKING A GOOD SHOE

Quality control in the shoe business is highly variable. When checking the forefoot flexion point of a shoe it is not uncommon for one shoe to flex at the ball of the foot and the other to flex pathologically farther back into the arch of the foot. If this shoe is truly desired then get another box out of that model and color and test it for function. If it passes and flexes at the ball of the foot correctly, then put the good functional shoes together and send back the pathological shoes for someone else to buy.

If enough of us do this the shoe stores may start checking their shoes and send them back for better quality control.

TESTING SHOES

- Take the insoles out and place your foot orthotic's in the shoes.
- Compare styles by wearing a different shoe on each foot and then walk and run in them.
- Continue this process with different models until the best two are found. The choice at this point should be cosmetic. Which one matches your school colors or clothes.

CHAPTER SEVENTEEN

ORTHOTICS AND SHOES

You have just learned how to correct foot subluxations, which tremendously helps foot mechanics. However, if the foots structure, when totally corrected, is still not within normal ranges of motion to the ground and leg, it will probably benefit from a foot orthotic.

That orthotic should go into a quality shoe that has a firm heel counter that will support the calcaneus. The mid sole of the shoe should be supportive with most of the flexion occurring at the location of the metatarsal heads. The mid foot should feel support on each side, while the metatarsal heads and toes should have a roomy toe box.

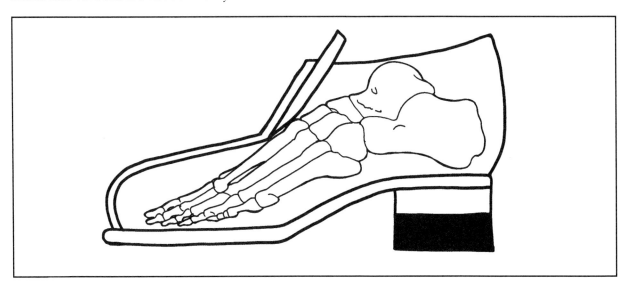

ORTHOTIC DEFINITIONS (2. p.14)

- FOOT ORTHOTIC- A device used to correct or accommodate certain foot abnormalities.
- FUNCTIONAL ORTHOTICS: Requirements.
  1. Support the foot so that the subtalar joint will function around neutral position.
  2. Allow normal motions in their proper sequence and eliminate abnormal/compensatory motions.
  3. Conform to all contours of the foot that help function.
  4. Be comfortable within a two week period.
  5. Be capable of being adjusted.

ACCOMODATIVE ORTHOTICS

- Any orthotic device that does not attempt to establish foot function around neutral subtalar position (or that restricts motion from the proper sequence.) (KGH)

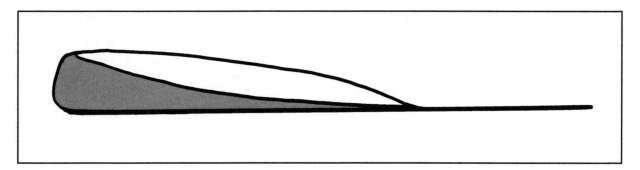

POSTS

- Wedges which are added to the orthotic (rearfoot, forefoot or both), to control the alignment of the foot and reduce excessive abnormal motion at the subtalar joint.
- They are designed to bring the ground up to the foots approach angle (neutral position) to the ground.

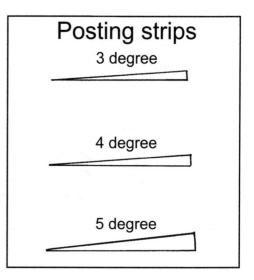

REAR FOOT VARUS POST

A medial wedge under the heel.

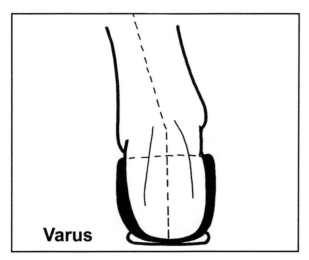

Lt Foot Before

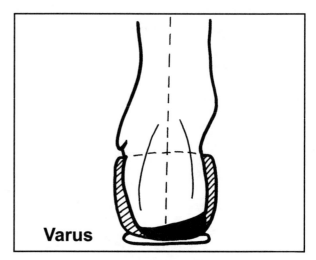

Lt. Foot After

FOREFOOT VARUS POST

A medial wedge under the metatarsal shafts usually posterior to the metatarsal heads.

Eighty six (86%) of the population has a varus foot.

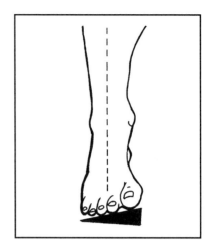

FOREFOOT VALGUS POST

A lateral wedge under the metatarsal shafts usually posterior to the metatarsal heads..

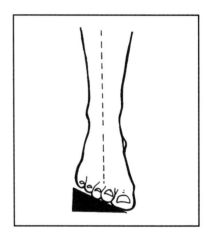

OTHER TYPES OF POSTS

- RIGID PLANTAR FLEXED 1ST RAY: A block under the 2nd through 5th metatarsal heads.
- RIGID DORSIFLEXED 1st RAY: A block under the first met head.
- EQUINUS: Add heel lift to exact height of limitation.
- CALCANEUS: Add sole forefoot lift with rocker bottom to improve stride.

ANKLE FOOT ORTHOSIS "AFO"

- A device that fits the leg and foot to control motion and create stability or function.
- It may be hinged or rigid.
- Types of uses may include "Drop Foot", "Unstable Ankle" or foot.

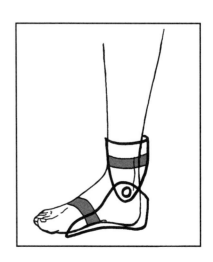

CHAPTER EIGHTEEN

FEET EXAM

- The following exam form is one developed in my clinic over the years. Information gathered on this form will help identify the underlying causes of many conditions and lead to a better diagnosis and treatment.
- The beauty of this form is the comparison of information from previous exams as the old orthotics wear out or new types or styles of orthotics are sought out. I can see the changes made in the feet. This information lets me know how well I accomplished the intended effect.

AVOID PIT FALLS BY

- Doing a thorough exam of the feet.
- Correct foot subluxations to restore normal glide of joints.
- Scan, cast or mold to a normal foot instead of a pathological foot.
- Prescribe to the lab the angles you expect to be in each foot orthotic. By law they must fill your prescription accurately.
- Make the orthotics yourself if it is an in house system.

ORTHOTIC EXAMINATION FORM

Patient Name: _____ Date: _____

SUPINE:

1. Observation:
   A. Anomalies
   B. Bunions
   C. Calluses
   F. Fungus
   H. Hammer Toe
   W. Wart

Top   Bottom

Right   Left   Right   Left

---

2. **Dorsiflexion Press Test** - Restricted: Left   Right

3. **Neutral Position:**   Left   Right
   Talus Head: Lateral   Medial   Lateral   Medial

ORTHOTIC POSTING				
LT	RT	Forefoot	Varus	Valgus
LT	RT	Rearfoot	Varus	Valgus

---

4. **Fixed Joints**   "X"

5. **Hypermobile Joints**   "O"

6. **Muscle Test:**

	Left		Right	
	Pre	Post	Pre	Post
Ant. Tibial	___	___	___	___
Post. Tibial	___	___	___	___
Peroneus Brev.	___	___	___	___
Peroneus Lng.	___	___	___	___

7. **FHL**   Left   Right

Anterior

Middle

Posterior

Left   Right

STANDING:

1. Longitudinal Arch: Left   (Flat   Low   Normal   High)
                          Right   (Flat   Low   Normal   High)

2. Achilles Tendon Apex   Left   Right
                          Lateral   Medial   Medial   Lateral

---

PRONE:

   Left   Forefoot: Varus   Valgus   Right   Forefoot: Varus   Valgus
          Rearfoot: Varus   Valgus   Rearfoot: Varus   Valgus

113

OBSERVATION OF BOTTOM OF SHOE VS FEET

There is a hundred times more information on the bottom of the feet than on the bottom of the shoe. Just observe and feel the skin and it tells a story much more thorough than a shoe, especially a newer shoe.

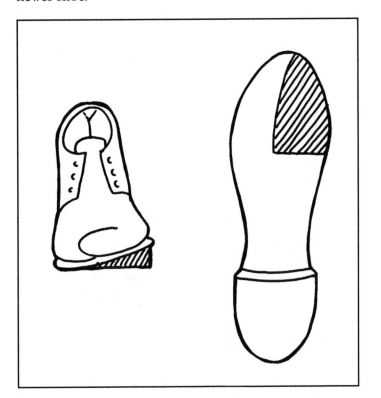
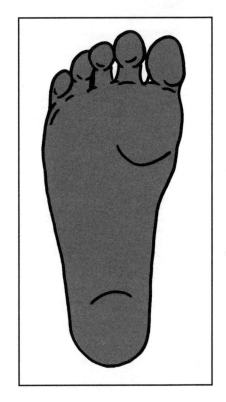

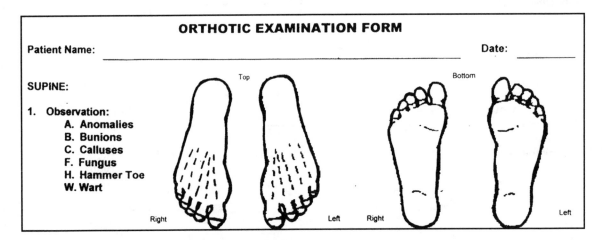

"Energy goes where energy flows" and energy stops where energy flops.

A great example of this is friction creates calluses. Look at and feel the bottom of the foot. Where there are calluses the foot is in contact with the ground. Where there is baby skin, the foot is not in contact with the ground. The feet automatically show where the patient is or is not walking and bearing weight.

114

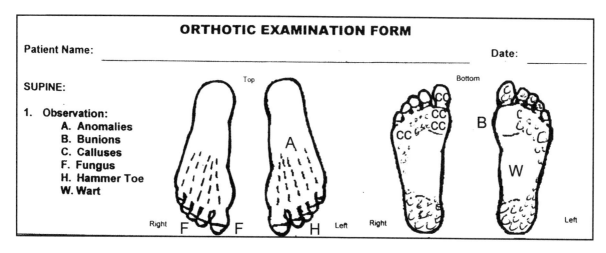

ORTHOTIC EXAMINATION FORM

Patient Name: _____ Date: _____

SUPINE:

1. Observation:
   A. Anomalies
   B. Bunions
   C. Calluses
   F. Fungus
   H. Hammer Toe
   W. Wart

Example of how to mark calluses and other anomalies of the feet.

40% of the forefoot calluses should be under the 1st MTP. The 5th MTP should be bearing 20% and the rest spread among the 2nd – 4th MTP's.

Joints that do not glide normally are fixated and marked with an "X".
Joints that glide excessively are hypermobile and marked with an "O".
Muscle tests are performed for foot function. FHL function is tested.

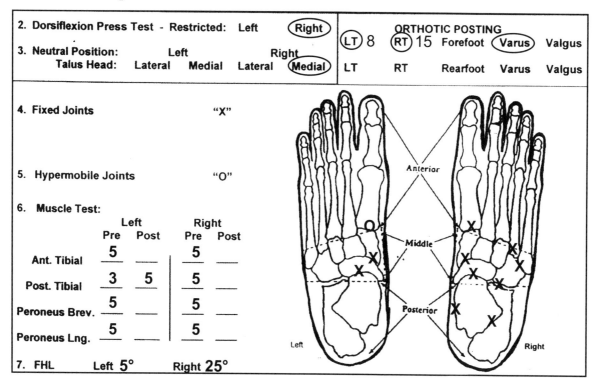

2. Dorsiflexion Press Test - Restricted: Left   (Right)

3. Neutral Position: Left   Right
   Talus Head: Lateral   Medial   Lateral   (Medial)

ORTHOTIC POSTING
(LT) 8   (RT) 15   Forefoot (Varus) Valgus
LT   RT   Rearfoot   Varus   Valgus

4. Fixed Joints   "X"

5. Hypermobile Joints   "O"

6. Muscle Test:

	Left Pre	Left Post	Right Pre	Right Post
Ant. Tibial	5		5	
Post. Tibial	3	5	5	
Peroneus Brev.	5		5	
Peroneus Lng.	5		5	

7. FHL   Left 5°   Right 25°

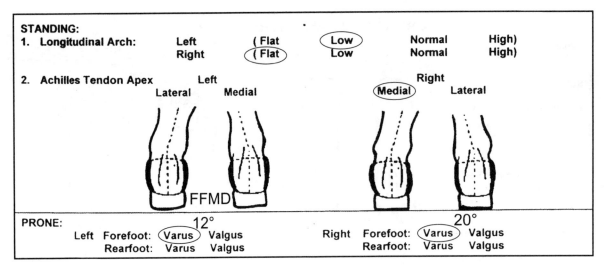

STANDING:

1. Longitudinal Arch:	Left	(Flat	Low	Normal	High)	
	Right	(Flat	Low	Normal	High)	

2. Achilles Tendon Apex

Left — Lateral / Medial   Right — (Medial) / Lateral

FFMD

PRONE:

Left Forefoot: (Varus) 12° Valgus   Right Forefoot: (Varus) 20° Valgus
Rearfoot: Varus Valgus   Rearfoot: Varus Valgus

I use the distal phalanx of my middle finger to determine longitudinal arch height.

If I cannot place the tip under the arch – the arch is flat.

If I can get half of the distal phalanx under the arch – the arch is low.

If I can get under to the distal joint space – the arch is normal.

If I can flex my distal phalanx under the arch – the arch is high.

Neutral position is documented by degrees with a FFMD.

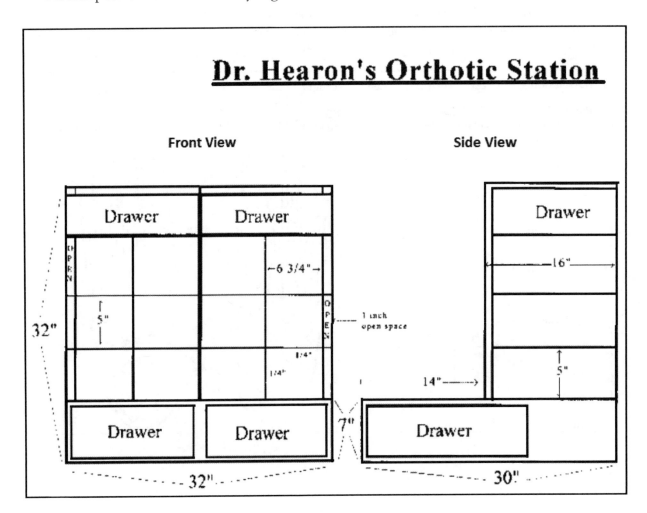

Dr. Hearon's Orthotic Station

Front View   **Side View**

FRONT VIEW OF ORTHOTIC STATION

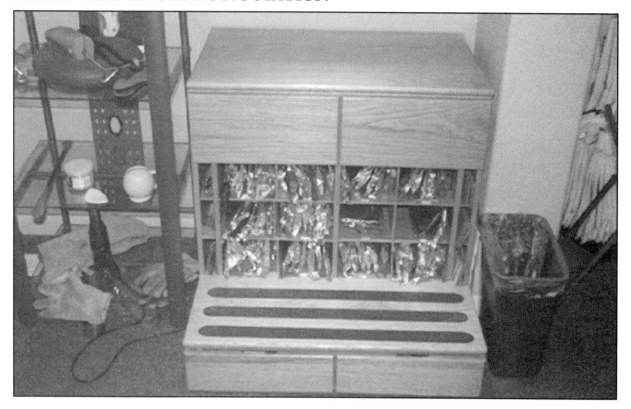

SIDE VIEW OF ORTHOTIC STATION

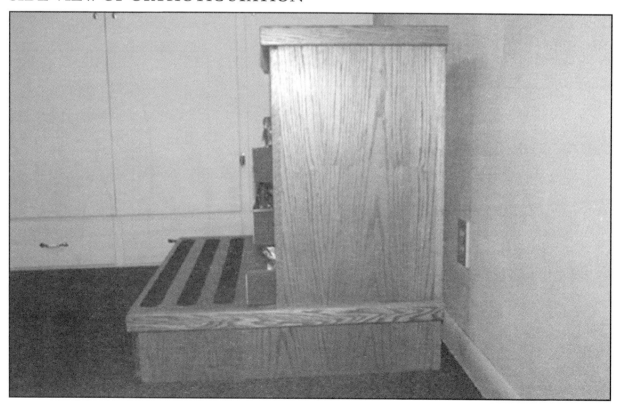

CHAPTER NINETEEN

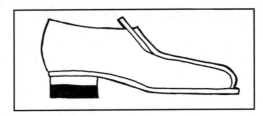

FEET ABNORMALITIES, HEEL LIFTS AND SHORT LEGS

HOW TO DETERMINE WHEN TO APPLY AN ORTHOTIC OR HEEL LIFT ON A CHILD OR ADULT.

Copyright 2009 Kevin G. Hearon

YOUR CHILD WILL GROW OUT OF IT

- This seems to be the standard answer most parents are given by well meaning doctors.
- The children acquired this from somewhere and it is more than likely it is from the parent that is in the room with you and the child.
- I would then ask the parent if they have any issues with their feet or the spouse that is not there in the room.

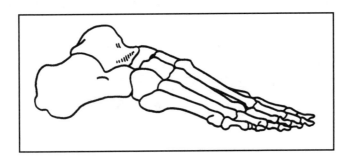

DID YOU GROW OUT OF IT?

- Usually the parent then tells a story of having to wear special shoes or of difficulty with their feet growing up.
- They explain how it has affected their life and how they have adapted to their feet issues and they are still dealing with them to this day.

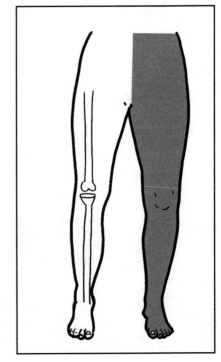

IF YOU DIDN'T GROW OUT OF IT, THEN WHY DO YOU EXPECT YOUR CHILD TO?

- Of course the standard answer is
- " because the doctor said so".
- It is at this moment the light bulb comes on in the parents mind and the shock of considering that the other doctors may have missed a key opportunity to help them.
- Now they move into the next logical question, because it is obvious their child has not "grown out of it".

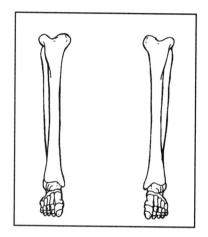

WHAT SHOULD I DO?

- This can be a very awkward moment depending upon the age of the child.
- The earlier the intervention usually the more that can be done to mold the growing bones into a better position of alignment.
- If the child is older the parents can feel robbed of the opportunity they had and did not know it.

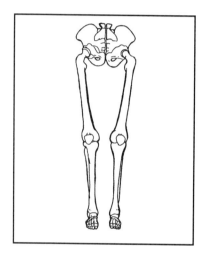

THIS DEPENDS UPON THE OSSIFICATION TIMES OF THE BONES

- As the bones change from cartilage to bone in the feet they respond to stress and adapt to the forces put upon them. This just follows the Laws of Healing in the bone responding to the Piezo-electric Effect which in the body is known as Wolff's Law.

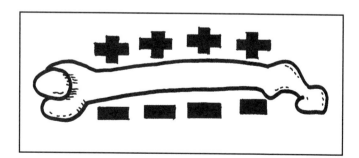

OSSIFICATION OF TODDLERS'S BONES

The talus, calcaneus, cuboid and navicular bones are key in their support for normal gait development. Some of the growth changes do not occur in the centers of the bones cartilaginous anlage [ahn-lah-guh] or any one axis but proceed eccentrically in different orientations.

Anne M. Hubbard[1]
James S. Meyer[1]
Richard S. Davidson[2]
Soroosh Mahboubi[1]
M. Patricia Harty[1]

Relationship Between the Ossification Center and Cartilaginous Anlage in the Normal Hindfoot in Children:
Study with MR Imaging

(30) AJR 1993; 161: 849-853

FOOT OSSIFICATION APPEARANCES

GRAY'S ANATOMY 35TH BRITISH EDITION OSTEOLOGY P.383

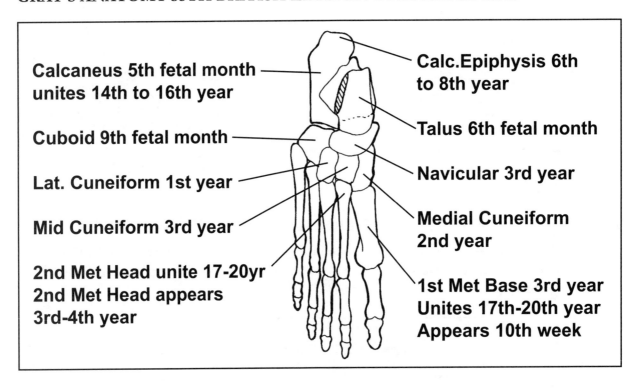

Calcaneus 5th fetal month unites 14th to 16th year

Cuboid 9th fetal month

Lat. Cuneiform 1st year

Mid Cuneiform 3rd year

2nd Met Head unite 17-20yr 2nd Met Head appears 3rd-4th year

Calc.Epiphysis 6th to 8th year

Talus 6th fetal month

Navicular 3rd year

Medial Cuneiform 2nd year

1st Met Base 3rd year Unites 17th-20th year Appears 10th week

INFANT UP TO TWO

- When an infant starts walking it is typical for them to pronate and have flat feet and some foot flair. The medial arch ossification appears/starts in the 3rd year to begin stability in the arch.
- It is not typical to be severely pigeon toed or duck feet after the age of two.
- At two years I recommend the child be brought in for evaluation because it is much easier to treat them early to get results quickly.

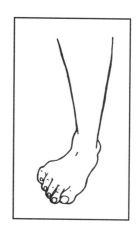

TWO TO FOUR

- It is important to check the children by the age of four. At this age it is much easier to respond to foot adduction or abduction issues with "gait plates".
- What gait plates do is counter the tibial and femoral torsion of the legs and feet so the child has a gait that is much closer to straight.
- The gait plate moves the foot into a position that de-rotates the foot and therefore the tibia and femur.

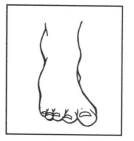

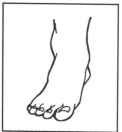

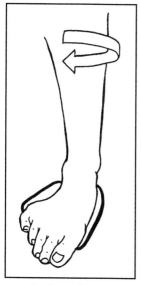

GAIT PLATES

Gait plates are placed under the metatarsal heads and can be full length to hold this position during ambulation.

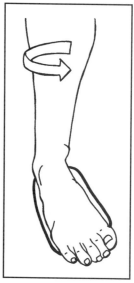

A plate that raises the lateral side of the foot twists the tibia and femur externally

A plate that raises the medial side of the foot twists the tibia and femur internally

121

GAIT PLATE DURATION

As the two to four year old wears these gait plates over the next three to six months, tibial and femoral torsion will decrease and the patient will tend to walk straight ahead.

At this point the gait plate may be taken out and the patient allowed to walk normally while observing for any changes over the next few months. Conventional foot orthotics may be in order if further control is needed.

DUCK FEET OR PIGEON TOED

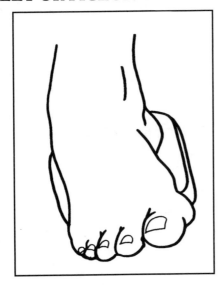

Duck feet post   Pigeon toed post

These angles start conservative and are increased
until a close to straight gait is attained.

DEGREES OF ANGULATION

- Please understand that the pictures and illustrations are exaggerated for simplification of the concept. The orthotics will be full length and narrower than appears in the drawing and tapered thinner at the met heads. I will frequently post the insole material or make a foam insole and post it.
- Most of these gait plates will be somewhere between 3 degrees to 10 degrees.
- The idea is to add posting strips and check the gait on the patient as you work toward getting the feet pointed straight ahead.

SOLE OF SHOE POSTING WOULD CORRECT DUCK FEET

This external way of doing gait plates is also an option which would be done by the shoe cobbler or certified pedorthist.

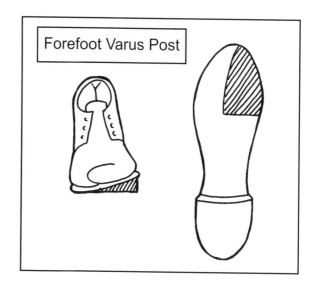

Forefoot Varus Post

FOUR TO EIGHT YEAR OLDS

- The difference is time for this age group when using the gait plates.
- This group may take six months to nine months to respond and straighten.
- Children do not seem to react to these like an adult would and usually adapt well due to the flexibility of the growth plates.

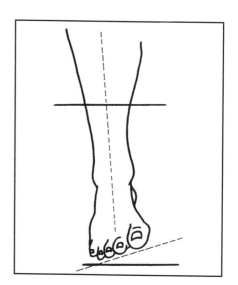

EIGHT TO TWELVE YEAR OLDS

- The difference is more time for this age group when using the gait plates.
- This group may take six months to a year to respond and straighten.
- Initially I see them a week after I first fit them and if they are doing good, I will see them in another two weeks
- It is a great idea to check them every two months for a year once you know they have adapted.

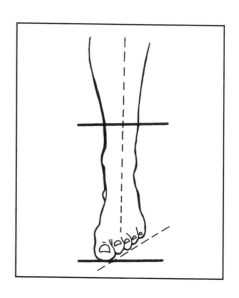

AGE 12 AND OLDER

- I will typically treat these youngsters as adults because the ossification does not lend itself to a timely result using gait plates.
- This age group is usually looking for performance and fitness benefits that they can feel quickly and relieve the stress they may feel in their feet, knees, hips and low back.

(16) Eslami M, et al. Effect of foot orthoses on magnitude and timing of rearfoot and tibial motions, ground reaction force and knee moment during running. J Sci Med Sport (2008), doi:10.1016/j.jsams.2008.05.001

(32) Resolution of Chronic Back, Leg and Ankle Pain Following
    Chiropractic Intervention and the Use of Orthotics
    Robert B. Mattson, D.C.1 J. Vertebral Subluxation Res. March

- When making foot orthotics for older children and adults it is important to know that the orthotics are only good if you wear them. Changes in economy of gait decline with time, usually by a month, if not supported most of the time.

(49) Changes in Gait Economy Between Full-Contact Custom-made Foot Orthoses and Prefabricated Inserts in Patients with Musculoskeletal Pain A Randomized Clinical Trial Leslie C. Trotter, DC, MBA, MSc, CPed (C)* Michael Raymond Pierrynowski, PhD†
    www.japmaonline.org/content/98/6/429.abstract 8-15-2011

- Treatment of low back pain utilizing the treatment of the feet by using custom made foot orthotics can reduce the symptoms and the duration of treatment by half according to research in the Journal of the American Podiatric Medical Association.
- When chiropractors utilize functional foot orthotics along with chiropractic care this should improve relief and healing time even more.

(11) Chronic low-back pain and its response to custom-made foot orthoses HJ Dananberg and M Guiliano, Journal of the American Podiatric Medical Association, Vol 89, Issue 3 109-117, 1999

LEG LENGTH AND HEEL LIFTS.

This is an area with much controversy and many approaches. As a result I will share with you what I have found works in my practice over decades of practice.

I hope this rings true to your logical mind and I especially hope it helps you in evaluating when to apply a heel lift and how much.

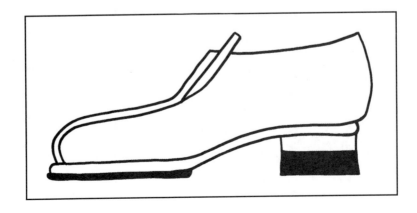

OLD MEASUREMENTS

- It is generally agreed that measuring the Internal malleoli to iliac crests and umbilicus leaves much to be desired.
- It does not show sacral unleveling.
- It cannot see the direction or rotation of the lumbar curve.

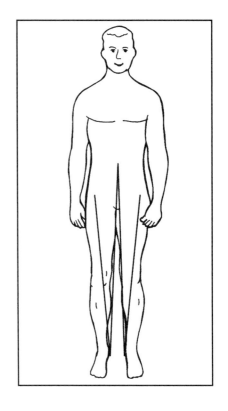

X-RAY SET UP

- To take a good anatomical X-ray it helps to understand the pitfalls that prevent a consistent and accurate film of the lumbar spine and pelvis.
- Most doctors that take spine x-rays do not consider, even in research, the many anatomical variations that the feet contribute to the height and length of the legs.
- It is important to look for a short calcaneus with one having a much smaller size. Look at the malleoli to see if they are even.
- Is there a tibia varum (bow leg) on one side and a rectus tibia on the other?
- Is one foot pronated (shorter) and the other supinated (taller) while standing? This will torque the pelvis toward the side of the supinated foot.
- Does the patient need an artificial assist to hold position?

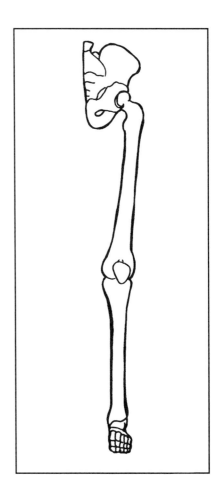

EFFECTS OF FEET POSITION TO HEIGHT
THE FOOT IS TALLER IN SUPINATION

PRONATION:

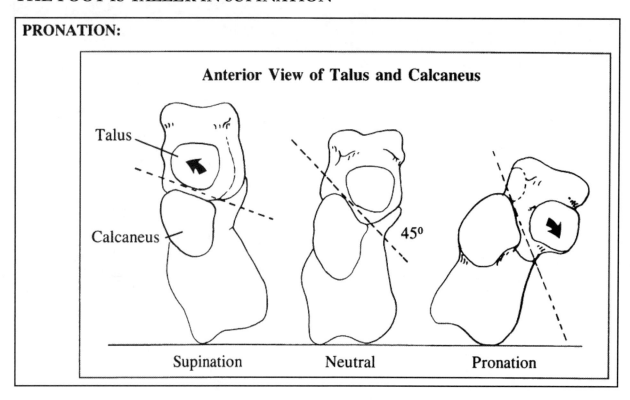

Anterior View of Talus and Calcaneus

Talus

Calcaneus

45°

Supination   Neutral   Pronation

HEIGHT DIFFERENCE

- The first thing you should notice is that there is a height difference of the calcaneus and talus in supination and pronation.
- So if someone taking an X-ray of the lumbo-sacral spine has one foot pronated and the other supinated it would affect leg length.

Supinated   Pronated

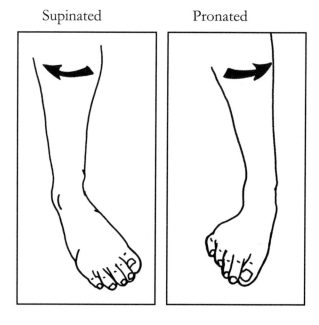

ARCH HEIGHT AFFECTED BY PRONATION AS WELL AS LENGTH OF FOOT.

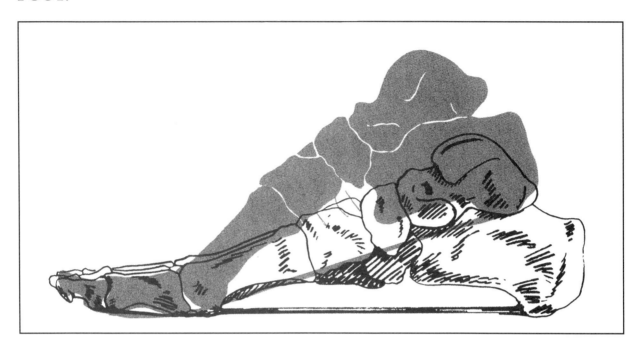

KNEE Q-ANGLE

- Pronation increases the Q-Angle of the knee and therefore shortens the leg.
- This lowers the hip on the same side.

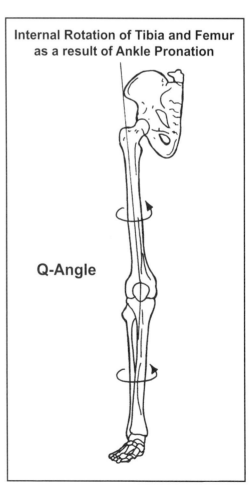

Internal Rotation of Tibia and Femur as a result of Ankle Pronation

Q-Angle

PRONATION LOWERS HIP

- This tilts the pelvis down on the same side due to the pull of the iliac muscle.
- This leans the lumbar spine toward this side due to the pull of the psoas muscle on the lumbar spine.

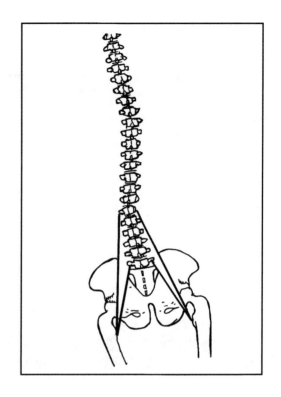

PATIENT POSITIONING CONCLUSION

- Foot position affects leg length.
- Ankle position affects leg length.
- Knee position affects leg length.
- Hip position affects leg length.
- Pelvis position affects leg length.
- With so many things affecting leg length, how do you take an X-Ray and control them to get an accurate measurement?

FEET CONTROL THE MECHANICS

- It is important at this point to remember that the feet control the kinetic chain of motion up the leg into the hip, pelvis and low back.
- When you control the feet, you control what's above them.
- It takes discriminating knowledge to address and eliminate many variable factors to take as accurate a film as possible.

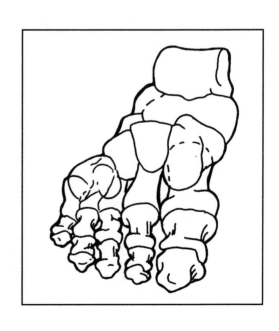

X-RAY POSITIONING OF PATIENT

I take an lumbo-sacral X-Ray of them standing with their feet shoulder wide apart, equally weighted and toes pointed straight ahead. I then get on the floor and check their arch height and ankle position and cause them to be identical. This is when I shoot the X-Ray.

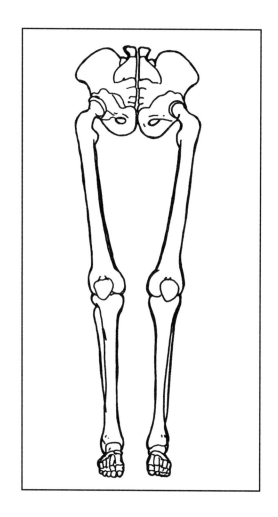

LINE MEASUREMENTS

- Taking a parallel from the edge of the film, draw these lines.
- Ischium
- Hip
- Sacral Base with both ends vertical over the femoral heads.
- Iliac Crest

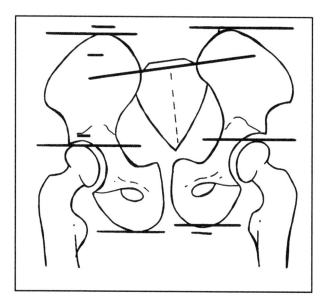

L/S X-RAY WITH LINES

Notice the lt. hip is 11mm lower but the lt. sacrum is only 2mm low and the spine is fairly straight. No lift needed.

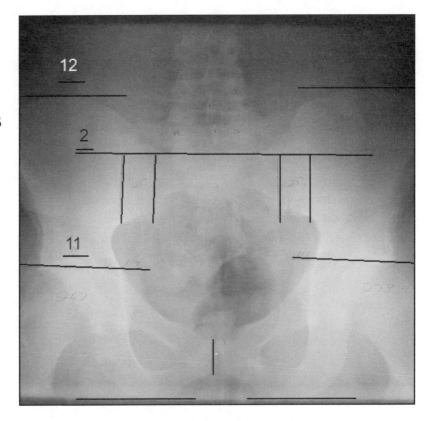

LT SHORT LEG & SACRUM

- This patient has both a short leg of 36mm and a low sacrum with a significant left lumbar curve.
- A left heel lift of 15mm is the starting point.
- How far down is the sacrum tilted over the femoral heads.

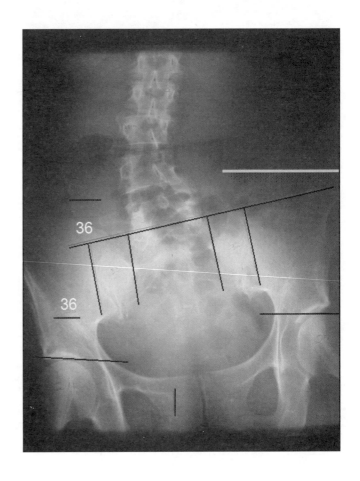

LT SHORT LEG OF 18MM

- 33 y/o female
- Lt short sacrum of 16mm.
- Lt short leg of 16mm.
- Mild lumbar curve to Lt.
- Heel lift of 6mm

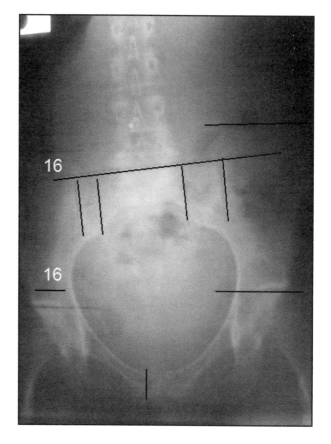

EXAMPLE OF DATA IN FILE ABOUT FILMS

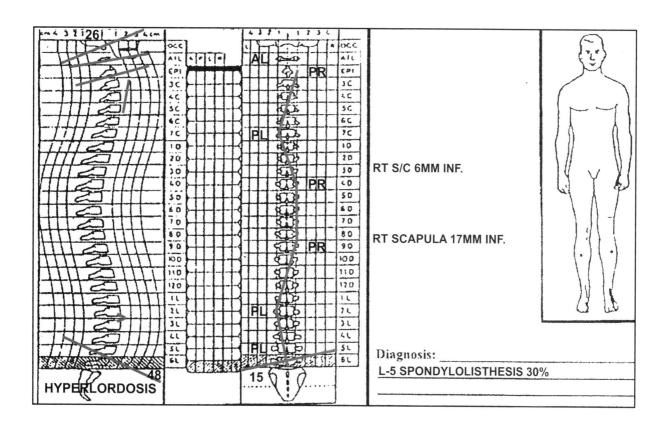

RT S/C 6MM INF.

RT SCAPULA 17MM INF.

Diagnosis: _____

L-5 SPONDYLOLISTHESIS 30%

HYPERLORDOSIS

SHORT LEG NEEDING NO HEEL LIFT

- The lt. leg is 8mm shorter than rt.
- The sacrum is 11mm lower on the lt. The line is drawn through the sacral notches vertical to each femoral head apex.
- The spine is straight.

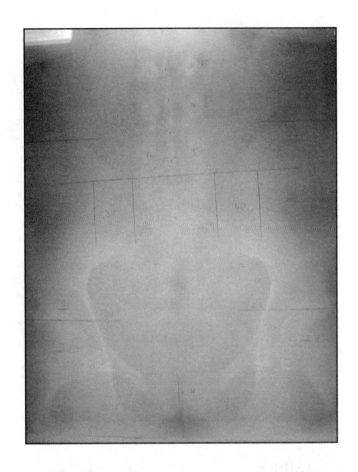

SHORT LEG AND SACRUM NEEDS HEEL LIFT OF 6MM

- The lt. leg is 15mm lower than the rt.
- The lt. sacrum is 12mm lower on the lt.
- The lumbar spine is curved to the lt.

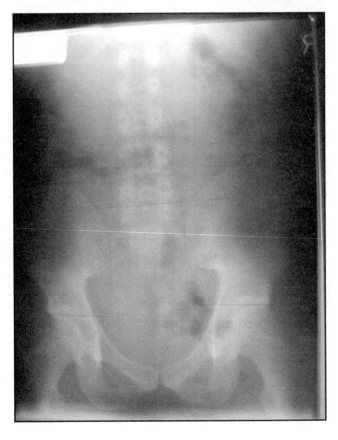

DOCUMENTATION OF KEY INFORMATION

- I like to put my X-ray findings on my exam form while I am measuring on the films. This gives me a quick visual of the key information.
- I can write an X-ray report from the information on this form if it were necessary.

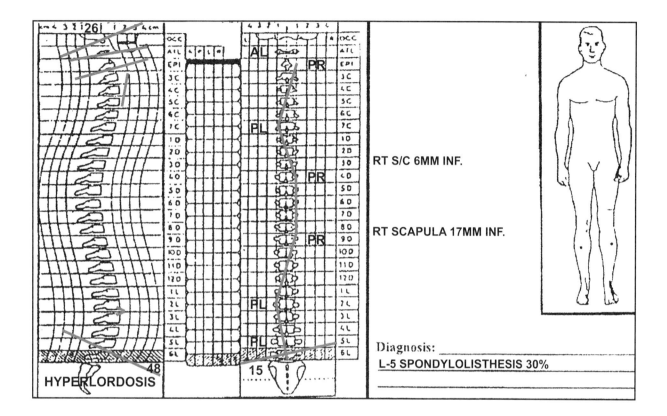

RT S/C 6MM INF.

RT SCAPULA 17MM INF.

Diagnosis: _____
L-5 SPONDYLOLISTHESIS 30%

HYPERLORDOSIS

FORMS ARE ON LINE

You can down load some of our forms by clicking on "Doctors Forms" at; kevinhearon.com; then go to Boise Sports icon

You are welcome to copy them and modify them for your use in your clinic.

You will find a letter of Medical Necessity for foot orthotics that is helpful to send with your forms to the insurance company.

LETTER OF MEDICAL NECESSITY

To Whom It May Concern:

The above referenced patient has been prescribed and fitted for bilateral functional foot orthotics for both dress and sport activities.

The medical condition of this patient produces considerable symptomatology affecting extremity function and spinal alignment. These controlling durable medical orthopedic appliances reduce foot deformation, toe malposition and osteoarthritic alterations in the joints of the feet, legs and spine. By managing this patient's condition with orthotics, the need for possible surgical intervention, equivocal post-surgical results, and revisional surgical procedures may be reduced or obviated. Biomechanical orthotics are used to obtain maximum normal function of the feet by aligning and retaining certain angular relationships between the various functional osseous segments. These are custom fabricated specifically for this patient and cannot be utilized by any other person.

There are additional components called post controls attached to the orthotics for the purpose of decreasing various force vectors of each muscle or muscle group. This improves the transfer of force through the feet and improves muscle dynamics. Attached is a claim for these orthotics.

If I may be of additional assistance with this matter, please do not hesitate to contact me.

In Good Health,

TRIAL PERIOD

- If you are undecided about prescribing a heel lift it may be better to wait and see how the patient does without one.
- Inform them that if the spine is not stable in three to four weeks they may need a heel lift.
- I prefer to begin on the side of conservative treatment with my patients.

THE TYPICAL APPLICATION OF LIFTS

- 1. Make the heel lift half of what the short leg or sacrum is. Short leg 12mm-heel lift 6mm.
- 2. Make the sole lift half of the heel lift.
- 3. Lift the side the spine leans toward.
- 4. Exactly level is not always the goal.
- 5. Wear the lifts almost always.
- 6. If the spine is not more stable in three to four weeks they may need a reevaluation.

HEEL & FOREFOOT LIFTS

- I only add a forefoot lift when the heel lift reaches ½" or 12mm.
- At this point I would prescribe a forefoot lift at half the heel lift height.
- A heel lift of half an inch (12mm) would get a quarter inch (6mm) forefoot lift.

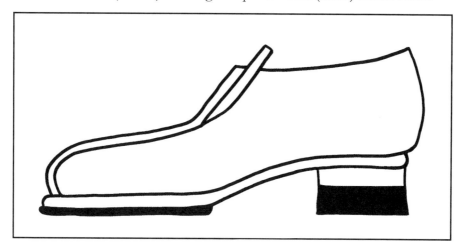

SUGGESTIONS TO GO BY

- Any forefoot varus or valgus correction greater than 15 degrees should go on the outside of the shoe usually.
- 15 degrees varus correction is usually enough for higher angled feet and can be worn for a while to see if it is enough
- If you need 20 degrees you could do 15 inside the shoe with an orthotic and 5 degrees more on the sole of the shoe.
- Any heel lift above ½" (12mm) should be applied to the external heel of the shoe.
- External heel lifts are always a good option for shoes no matter what height.

ADAPTING TIME

- I use the analogy of the athlete playing a new sport. The first week of training they are sore. The pet name they give is "Hell Week".
- By the second week it is usually less sore. If it has not improved some I will re-evaluate.
- By the third week they should be used to the activity and adapted well. If they are not very satisfied (80% better) by the third week then a modification of the orthotic is usually in order.

CONSISTENT IN WEARING

- It is important to inform the patient that wearing the orthotics at all times, the first three months, while weight bearing is critical for success.
- The feet will lock up again if they walk barefoot much except in sand.
- If they want to walk barefoot, it must be on their tippy toes because this locks the feet and prevents them from subluxating when out of the foot orthotics.
- After three months they can walk barefoot or without the orthotics for a few hours.

TAPING ASSISTS HEALING OF THE FEET

- Many years ago I learned about functional taping from Dr. Leroy Perry. The concepts of recreating the tendons, muscles and ligaments with Elasticon tape reestablished function and protection in an injured joint while still allowing motion within a safe physiologic envelope.
- Taping the foot is one of the ways I unload the plantar fascia and muscles of the plantar surface. My usual approach starts with a foot slipper and progresses from there if needed to assist the medial longitudinal arch.

(19) Tape That Increases Medial Longitudinal Arch Height Also Reduces Leg Muscle Activity: A Preliminary Study MELINDA FRANETTOVICH, 2, ANDREW CHAPMAN1,2, and BILL VICENZINO2 1Australian Institute of Sport, Canberra, AUSTRALIA; and 2University of Queensland, Brisbane, AUSTRALIA

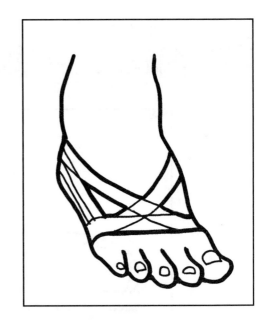

SOFT SAND WALKING

- The one place most people say they love to walk is on a sandy beach.
- This is understandable because the sand absorbs shock and conforms to the congenital angles and shape of the feet. Natural support occurs and it just feels naturally right.
- The intrinsic muscles of the feet get good functional exercise in the sand as they grasp and push.

CHAPTER TWENTY

6 PRINCIPLES OF THE FEET

- <u>If it's fixated – mobilize it:</u> The joints need to glide for shock absorption.
- <u>If it's hypermobile – stabilize it:</u> For ligaments to shorten they need firm support.
- <u>If it's normal – allow it's normal motion:</u> An orthotic should allow controlled pronation for shock absorption or set the foot up for conditioning to normal function.
- <u>Match the flexibility of the orthotic to the weight</u> and control needed by the feet for the activity that is stressing them. How many times body weight?
- <u>Determine the style of the orthotic</u> by matching the characteristic of the shoe it will be used for. e.g.- dress, casual, sport etc.
- <u>Consider the spatial condition of the shoe</u> being worn and can it tolerate a full length, sulcus length or ¾ length. eg- size of toe box, depth of shoe.

MULTIPLE STYLES

Ideally a person should have multiple sets of foot orthotics that control forces while walking (1 to 3x body weight), or running (3 to 5x body weight), and jumping (5 to 7x body weight). The varying strengths of the orthotics would attenuate shock more efficiently and control the accumulated load of the kinetic chain within safer limits. The idea is to keep the healing rate higher than the irritation rate. It is nice to change into a fresh orthotic after a workout.

AVOID PIT FALLS BY

- Doing a thorough exam of the feet.
- Correct foot subluxations to restore normal glide of joints.
- Scan, cast or mold to a normal foot instead of a pathological foot.
- Prescribe to the lab the angles you expect to be in each foot orthotic, or make them yourself if it is an in house system.

CHOOSING AN ORTHOTIC

The analogy I like to use with a patient is the difference between a truck, family car and a sports car.

TRUCK; The truck has a lot of space and can carry a big load much like most athletic shoes. It is usually full length that is thicker and firmer to handle the heavier load of forces during competition.

FAMILY CAR; The family car is moderate in size and thinner. It can be full length or ¾ length depending upon toe box volume. It has medium resistance and is useful for the daily errands of the casual shoe.

SPORTS CAR; The sports car is small and sleek with confined space and fits into those narrow tight patent leather dress shoes, soccer shoes, bike shoes, ballet slippers or ice skates. It is usually ¾ length to allow for a very tight toe box. Strength of resistance depends upon the activity it is used for.

DENSITY OF ORTHOTIC WHEN WALKING

VERY FLEXIBLE: For diabetics or people under 50 lbs.

FLEXIBLE: For easy comfort and people 50 to 100 lbs.

FIRM FLEXIBLE: Moderate control and people 100 to 150 lbs.

FIRM: Moderately firm control and people 150 to 200lbs.

SEMI RIGID: Solid control of higher forces for the 200 to 250lbS.

RIGID: Supporting the 250 to 300 lb. person.

VERY RIGID: The heavy weight control for the 300 + lb. person.

These densities will increase with running and jumping.

The average typical malc has a grip strength of 80 to 140 lbs. so a firm density orthotic will feel quite strong when testing its deformation. Therefore a firm orthotic will feel rigid to you probably.

FOOT CAPTURE METHODS EVALUATED

TWO DIMENSIONAL FOOT PRESSURE SCANS ON FLAT SURFACES WHETHER IT BE DIGITAL OR INK ON PAPER ARE NOT GOOD INDICATERS OF MEDIAL LONGITU-DINAL ARCH HEIGHT.

THE PUBLIC SHOULD BE AWARE THAT THESE APPROACHES TO CAPTURING THE FEET ARE BASICALLY ONLY GOOD FOR LENGTH AND WIDTH BUT NOT HEIGHT OF THE ARCH.

EVEN IF THE INSTRUMENT CAPTURES FORCES ON THE BOTTOM OF THE FEET, IT CANNOT GIVE ACCURATE ARCH HEIGHT.

(36) J Am Podiatr Med Assoc. 2006 Nov-Dec;96(6):489-94.

Use of plantar contact area to predict medial longitudinal arch height during walking.

McPoil TG, Cornwall MW.

CHAPTER TWENTY ONE

TYPES OF FOOT CAPTURE SYSTEMS I USE
THAT COULD BE USED IN A CLINIC.

- Injection mold orthotics – made in house to the patient in about twenty minutes.
- 3D scan of the feet down loaded electronically to the lab to be cut out by a CAD (computer aided drafting) mill and returned 4 days later.
- Foam cast orthotics sent to a lab of your choice with varying types of topography capture and return time from days to weeks.
- Generic and modifiable pre-shaped and heat molded orthotics of varying materials.

INJECTION MOLD ORTHOTICS

- From start to finish an experienced doctor can easily make an injection mold foot orthotic in about twenty minutes. The beauty of this method is the patient walks out with the orthotics in their shoes and is getting their correction immediately.
- The other thing I like is the total control over the process with the patient and I get to see the change in gait mechanics with immediate feedback from them.

INJECTION MOLD ORTHOTICS

Take the closed package of the size stated and press it to the foot of the patient. There should be a thumb width between the end of the toes and the end of the foot orthotic. In this way you can be sure of the correct size.

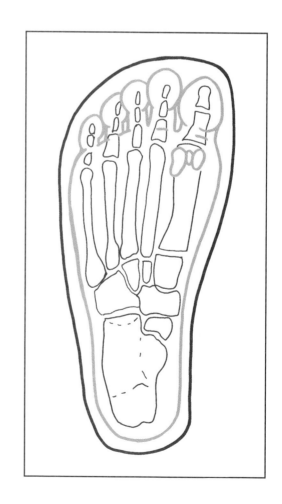

Take the insoles out of the shoes if you can.
See if the orthotics fit into the shoes.
Trim the forefoot area only if needed.
Do not cut into the black bladder area yet.
Cut and shape the posting strips to the orthotics.
Peel off the backing of the posting strips.
Do not apply the strips yet.
Get the injection syringes and roller ready.
Get a quarter cup of hot water.

INJECTION MOLD ORTHOTICS

Fill the syringe up to the cc the package says.

Open the flap on the orthotic and expose the injection hole and inject the hot water. Squeeze the orthotic and look for water out of the 3 escape holes. Close the flap.

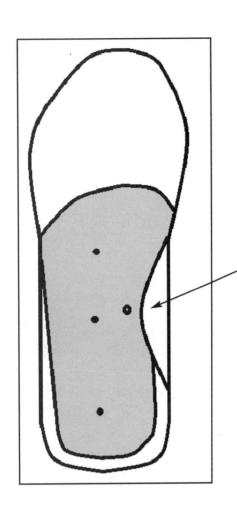

Injection hole

Apply the posting strip over the flap posterior to the met heads and use the roller to disperse the hot water in the orthotic. This should only take about 5 seconds to roll out.

The polymer resin in the orthotic will fill around 4 degrees of varus easily as it hardens. The posting strip will angle the rest of the correction.

Place the orthotic into the shoe and have the patient stand up on it and tie the shoe for the patient. The other foot should be on tip toes until it gets into the other orthotic.

Repeat the process for the other orthotic.

Now have the patient go for a five minute walk.
The orthotics are now 90% molded to the feet.
Take the orthotics out and remove the flaps.
Restore the posts to their position on orthotics.
You may now modify the orthotics further.
FHL cut outs can be made and trimming.

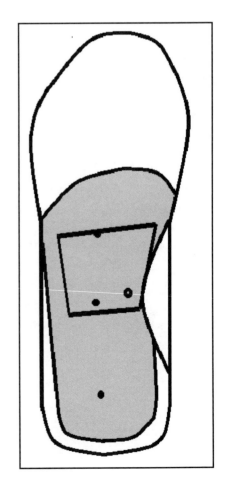

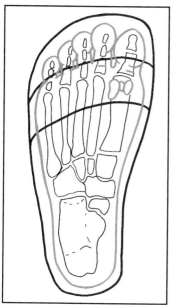

Orthotics can be cut to shorter lengths to accommodate to toe box room. Three lengths are typical – full length, sulcus length and ¾ length.

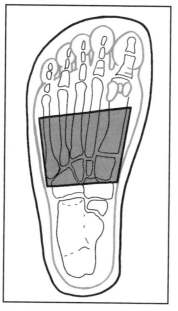

Correct positioning of the posts is important. The forefoot post should be posterior to the met heads. Posts will be from 3 to 10 degrees on the orthotic.

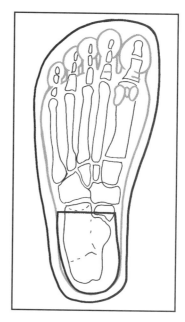

Rear foot posts should match the contour of the orthotic. They will be either 3 or 5 degrees.

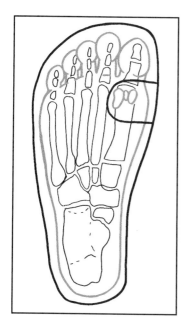

FHL cut outs should surround the sesamoid bones generously to allow plantar flexion of the 1st met head when under load.

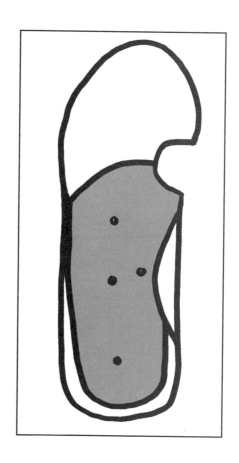

It has been my position for many years that usually when an orthoses is made well for the patients feet that they should feel much better by the third week of wearing them. I believe that if I have done my job well the patient should usually never want to go back to their old way of walking, running or riding. Now the research backs this up.

(51) The Short-term Effectiveness of Full-Contact Custom-made Foot Orthoses and Prefabricated Shoe Inserts on Lower-Extremity Musculoskeletal Pain

A Randomized Clinical Trial

Leslie C. Trotter, DC, MBA, MSc, CPed(C) * and Michael Raymond Pierrynowski, PhD

Journal of the American Podiatric Medical Association Volume 98 Number 5 357-363 2008

Copyright © 2008

3D SCAN ORTHOTICS

3D scan technology has come a long way and can be done with pins or laser. If you are prescribing over ten foot orthotics a month in your practice this may be a fit. The CAD mill can cut out the shape within a half millimeter accuracy of your foot I am told. Modifications can be done on the computer before sending the data to the lab. Turn around time is about four workdays. Technical minded people like this approach.

3D SCAN EQUIPMENT

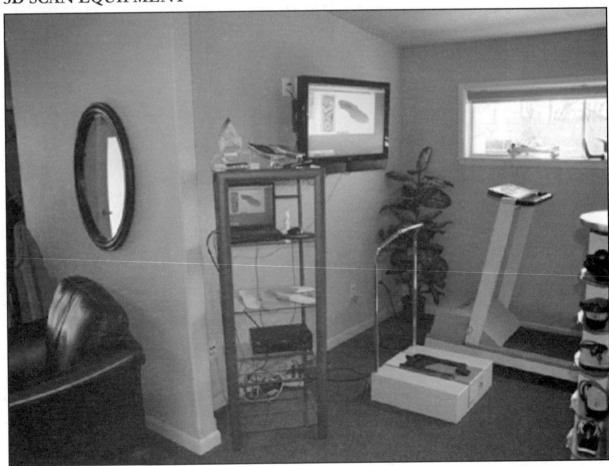

3D SCAN OF THE FOOT IN NEUTRAL

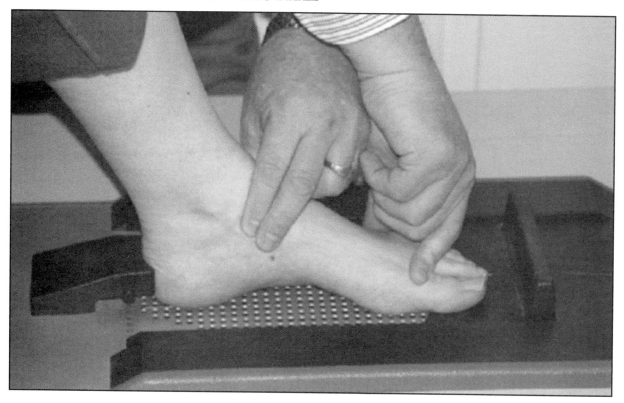

PINS HAVE CAPTURED THE SHAPE OF THE ARCH

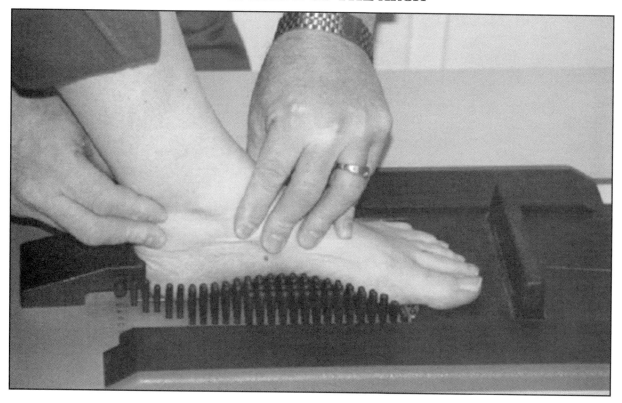

THIS IS NOW DIGITIZED AND SENT INTO A C.A.D. MILL TO BE CUT.

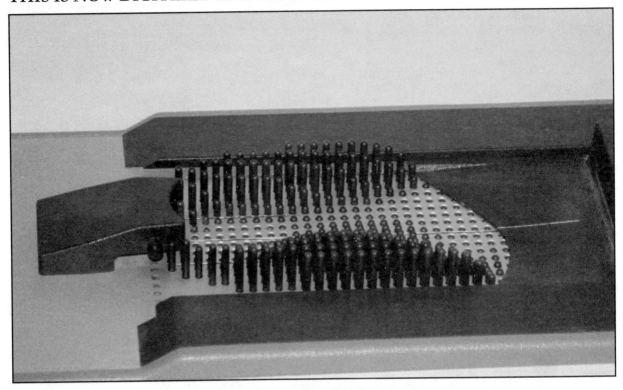

THE DIGITIZED PICTURE HAS COLOR VARIATIONS SHOWING HALF MILLIMETER INCREMENTS AND CAN BE MODIFIED BY THE DOCTOR ON THE COMPUTER.

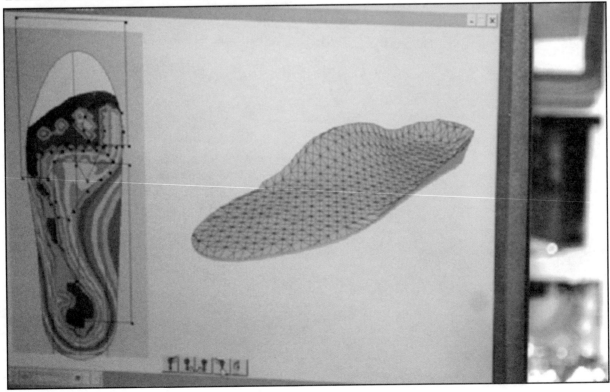

FOAM CAST ORTHOTICS

The difference between selling an orthotic and prescribing an orthotic is discriminating knowledge. By law the lab must fill your prescription. So if you give the lab the angles you want on each orthotic it better come back that way. Most feet are different and the orthotic should be different, not the same. If your lab keeps sending you identical orthotics, maybe it's time to switch labs. Checking the box "post to cast" is giving up your control. Take control and prescribe the angles you measured for your patient.

FOOT CASTING IN FOAM SHOULD BE DONE IN NEUTRAL POSITION.

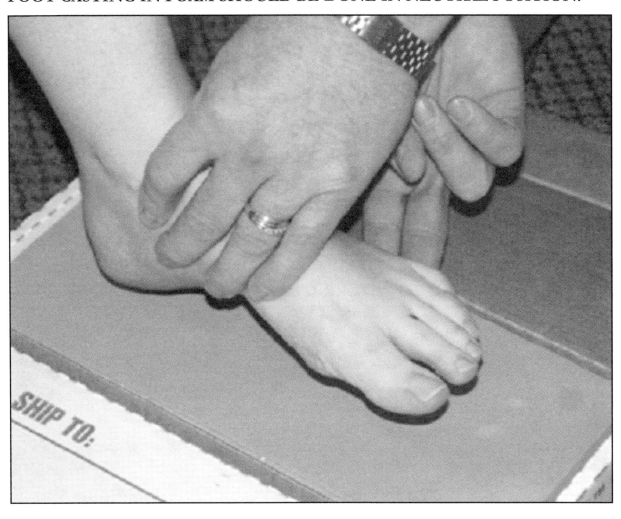

STABILIZING THE FOOT WHILE APPLYING PRESSURE IS IMPORTANT.

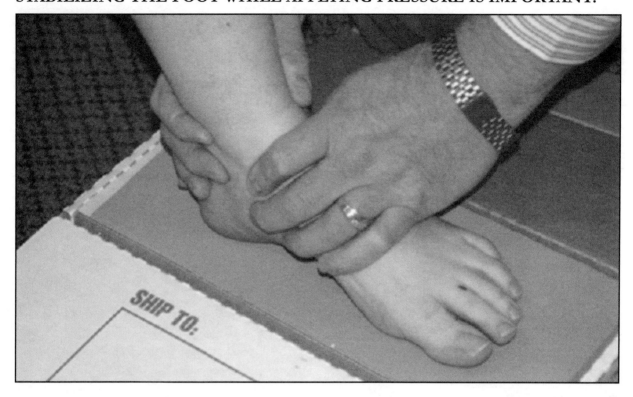

PRESSURE ON THE 4TH & 5TH MET HEADS HELPS CAPTURE THE NEUTRAL ANGLE. SOME PREFER NOT TO PERFORM THIS STEP.

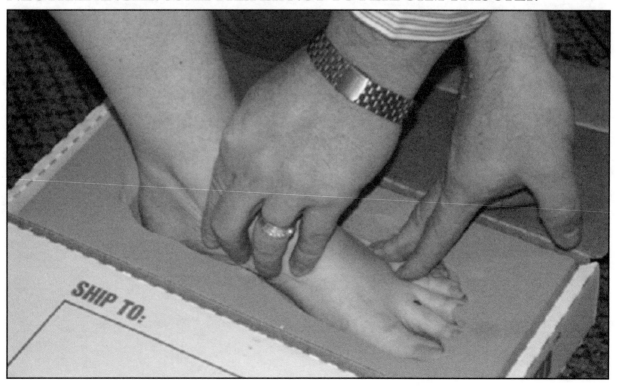

WHAT CASTING METHOD IS THE BEST?

There seems to be considerable controversy over which casting or capture method is the best and each group has pretty good reasons why they believe in the way they do it. There is even some research to show that maybe there is some parity in the reliability of different techniques.

The bottom line from a clinical standpoint is; Do the patients get well?

Personally I use a few different ways of casting and capturing neutral position. I inform the patient of the different approaches I use to cast or capture their feet and involve them in the decision. Each approach comes with a different companies orthotics.

(50) Ability of Foot Care Professionals to Cast Feet Using the Nonweightbearing Plaster and the Gait-Referenced Foam Casting Techniques

Leslie C. Trotter, DC, CPed(C), MBA * and Michael Raymond Pierrynowski, PhD

(J Am Podiatr Med Assoc 98(1): 14–18, 2008)

COMPARISON OF 3D DIGITAL CASTING VERSUS MANUAL FOAM CASTING OF THE FEET FOR THE DESIGN AND FABRICATION OF CUSTOM FOOT ORTHOSES

KEVIN G. HEARON, D.C., CCEP, CCSP

Conclusion: A statistical analysis (of 22 patients who underwent an examination and adjustment of the feet) demonstrated greater foot comfort and patient satisfaction from custom orthotics designed with the 3D digital casting technique over those designed using manual foam casting.

Journal of Vertebral Subluxation Research: January 31, 2008

GENERIC, MODIFIABLE AND HEAT MOLDED ORTHOTICS.

- Generic orthotics are frequently a low cost item that are the introductory choice of people initially trying to self diagnose and help their aching feet at usually a 4 degree varus angle.
- Modifiable orthotics can be changed intrinsically or extrinsically through either heat molding or external posting of its angle and shape. They vary in length, thickness, materials and strength of resistance.

APPLICATION OF THE MASTER CONTROL SYSTEMS

The combination of including the other Master Control System (the kinetic chain) from the ground up with powerful skills of the chiropractor treating the whole body through the nervous system from the top down is a strong formula for success.

Utilizing the ideas and concepts in this book as a practical approach and application in the practice of chiropractic will usually help stabilize many conditions that were previously over looked. More research is being done demonstrating the benefits of this approach.

(32) Resolution of Chronic Back, Leg and Ankle Pain Following Chiropractic Intervention and the Use of Orthotics Robert B. Mattson, D.C.1 J. Vertebral Subluxation Res. March 20, 2008 1

REFERRALS

It is important to remember when faced with a difficult and non-responsive patient, to utilize your fellow professionals in podiatry and orthopedics for their input and opinion. The interprofessional communication may diversify the options for the patient and clarify your position in the treatment of the condition.

CONCLUSION

The lower extremity is a magnificent kinetic chain working in either cooperation or conflict. The origin of the problems can come from either end of the lower extremity. The low back or pelvis may be subluxated and compromise nerve supply and mechanical function down the leg to the feet. Faulty shock absorption and increased joint stress will usually result.

When feet subluxate and loose normal mechanics they will frequently cause gait compensations that alter pelvic and low back dynamics.

All of the joints in the lower extremity and above it are affected in some way eventually if correction does not occur in a timely manner. A healthy skepticism is useful in tracking down mechanical and neurologic aberrations.

To truly fix the patient and prevent chronic recurring problems, we would do well to look at the lower extremity as part of our examination and treatment protocol.

REFERENCES

1. Astrom M, Arvidson T.: Alignment and joint motion in the normal foot. J Orthop Sports Phys Ther. 1995;22:216-222.

2. Bar, Aharon, Ph.D., Foot Biomechanics and Orthotic Therapy,, Orthofeet Inc. 1989.

3. Blauvelt, C. T., Nelson, Fred R. T. M.D., Orthopaedic Terminology, C.V. Mosby Co. 1985.

4. Buchanan KR, Davis I., The relationship between forefoot, midfoot, and rearfoot static alignment in pain-free individuals. J Orthop Sports Phys Ther. 2005;35:559-566.

5. Calliet, Rene M.D., Foot and Ankle Pain, F.A. davis Co. 1974.

6. Cambron et al. Shoe Orthotics for Low Back Pain, JMPT month 2011; Dynamic Chiropractic Vol. 28, Issue 07, March 26, 2010

7. Cuthbert S, Muscle Imbalance; The Goodheart and Janda models

8. Danenberg ,Howard J., D.P.M., Functional hallux Limitus and its Relation to Gait Efficiency, Journal of the American Podiatric Association, Volume 76, No. 11, November 1986.

9. Danenberg, Howard J., D.P.M., The Conservative Treatment of Hallux Limitus, Current Podiatric Medicine, April 1990.

10. Danenberg, Lawton, Dinapoli, Hallux Limitus and Non-Specific Gait Related Bodily Trauma, Podiatry Education & Research Institute Update 90, Reconstruction of the Foot and Leg, P. 52, 1990.

11. Danenberg HJ, Guiliano A, Chronic Low back pain and its Response to Custom Made Foot Orthoses. J Amer Pod Med Assoc Vol 89, Issue 3 109-117 1999

12. Daniels, L., M.A., Worthingham, C., Ph.D., Muscle Testing, W.B. Saunders Co. 1961.

13. Donatelli RA, Wooden MJ. F. A. Davis; Biomechanical orthotics. In: Donatelli RA, ed. The Biomechanics of the Foot and Ankle. Vol. 2. Philadelphia: 1996:255-279.

14. Donatelli R, Wooden M, Ekedahl SR, Wilkes JS, Cooper J, Bush AJ.: Relationship between static and dynamic foot postures in professional baseball players. J Orthop Sports Phys Ther. 1999;29:316-325; discussion 326-330.

15. Elveru RA, Rothstein JM, Lamb RL., Goniometric reliability in a clinical setting: subtalar and ankle joint measurements. Phys Ther. 1988;68:672-677.

16. Eslami M, et all, Effect of Foot Orthoses on Magnitude and Timing of Rearfoot and Tibial Motions Ground Reaction Force and Knee Moment During Running. J Sci Med Sport (2008) doi; 10.1016/JJsams.2008.05.001

17. Fick, D., Albright, J., Murray, B., Relieving Painful Shin Splints, The Physician and Sports Medicine, Vol. 20, No 12 December, 1992.

18. Friedman, Pregnancy, The Physician and Sports Medicine Vol. 18, No. 9, September 1990.

19. Franettovich M. et al, The ability to predict dynamic foot posture from static measurements. J Am Podiatr Med Assoc. 2007;97:115-120.

20. Franettovich M. et al, Tape That increases medial longitudinal arch height also reduces leg muscle activity. 1 Australian Institute of Sport, Canberra, Australia, and 2 University of Queensland, Brisbane, Australia.

21. Garbalosa JC, McClure MH, Catlin PA, Wooden M., The frontal plane relationship of the forefoot to the rearfoot in an asymptomatic population. J. Orthop Sports Phys Ther. 1994;20:200-206.

22. Glasoe, WM, Yack, HJ, Saltzman, CL,. Anatomy and Biomechanics of the First Ray. Phys. Ther. 1999; 79. 854-859.

23. Hamill J, Bates BT, Knutzen KM, Kirkpatrick GM.: Relationship between selected static and dynamic lower extremity measures. Clin Biomech. 1989;4:217-225.

24. Hartley, Anne, B.P.H.E., Practical Joint Assessment (A Sports Medicine Manual), Cat Mosby Year Book 1990.

25. Hearon, Kevin G., D.C., What You Should Know About Extremity Adjusting, self published, 1981. Now in its ninth edition.

26. Hearon KG, Advanced Principles of Lower Extremity Adjusting 2nd Edition Self published 1994

27. Hicks, J., The Mechanics of the Foot, Part II: The Plantar Aponeurosis and the Arch, J. Anat. 88: 25, 1954.

28. Hoppenfeld, Stanley M.D., Clinical Neurology, J.B. Lippincott Co. 1977.

29. Hoppenfeld , Stanley, M.D., Physical Examination of the Spine and Extremities, Appleton-Century-Crofts 1976.

30. Hubbard, AM. et al, Relationship between the ossification center and the cartilaginous anlage in the normal hind foot in children. AJR 1993; 161: 849-853.

31. Johansen, H. et. al., The Anterior Cruciate Ligament: A Sensor Acting on the Gamma Muscle Spindle Systems of Muscle Around the Knee Joint. Neuro-Orthopedics Vol. 9, P. 1-23, 1990.

32. Mattson, RB, Resolution of chronic back, leg and ankle pain following chiropractic intervention and the use of orthotics. D.C. 1, J Vert Sub Res. March 20, 2008 1

33. Mazion, J. M., Illustrated Manual of Neurological and Orthopedic Tests, Self Published 1980.

34. McPoil TG, Cornwall MW.: Relationship between three static angles of the rearfoot and the pattern of rearfoot motion during walking. J Orthop Sports Phys Ther. 1996;23:370-375.

35 . McPoil TG, Cornwall MW.: The relationship between static lower extremity measurements and rearfoot motion during walking. J Orthop Sports Phys Ther, 1996;24:309-314

36. McPoil TG, Cornwall MW.: Use of plantar contact area to predict medial longitudinal arch height during walking. J Am Podiatr Med Assoc. 2006 Nov-Dec. 96(6): 489-94

37. McPoil TG, Cornwall MW.: Prediction of dynamic foot posture during running using the longitudinal arch angle. J Am Podiatr Med Assoc. 2007;97:102-107.

38. Menz HB,: Two feet, or one person? Problems associated with statistical analysis of paired data in foot and ankle medicine.. Foot. 2004;14:2-5.

39. Miller, Kevin, "LCNC" Lateral Cuneiform Navicular Complex, e-mail 6-23-2011 .

40. Norkin CC, Levangie PK., Joint Structure & Function: A Comprehensive Analysis. 2nd ed. Philadelphia: F. A. Davis; 1992.

41. Portney LG, Watkins MP.: Foundations of Clinical Research: Applications to Practice. 2nd ed. Upper Saddle River, NJ: Prentice Hall; 2000.

42. Prithvi Raj, P., Practical Management of Pain, Year Book Medical Publishers Inc. 1986.

43. Root M, Orien W, Weed J. Clinical Biomechanics – Second Edition: Normal and Abnormal Function of the Foot. Vol. 2. Los Angeles: Clinical Biomechanics Corporation; 1977.

44. Sandberg R, et al, Operative versus non-operative treatment of recent injuries to the ligaments of the knee; J of Bone and Joint Surgery, Vol. 69A October 1987

45. Schafer, R. C., D.C., Chiropractic Management of Sports and Recreational Injuries, Williams and Wilkins 1982.

46. Schafer, R. C., D.C., Clinical Biomechanics: Musculoskeletal Actions and Reactions. Williams and Wilkins 1987.

47. Shultz and Villnave, Extremity Orthopedic Tests,. Self Published 1983

48. Smith LS, Clarke TE, Hamill CL, Santopietro F.: The effects of soft and semi-rigid orthoses upon rearfoot movement in running. J Am Podiatr Med Assoc. 1986;76:227-233.

49. Trotter LC, Pierrynowski MR, Changes in gait economy between full contact custom made foot orthoses and prefabricated inserts. J Am Podiatr Med Assoc. 2008 Nov-Dec; 98(6) 429-35

50. Trotter LC, Pierrynowski MR, Ability of foot care professionals to cast feet using the nonweight bearing plaster and the gait referenced foam casting techniques. J Am Podiatr Med Assoc 98(1): 14-18, 2008

51. Trotter LC, Pierrynowski MR, The short term effectiveness of full contact custom made foot orthoses and prefabricated shoe inserts on lower-extremity musculoskeletal pain. A randomized clinical trial. J Am Podiatr Med Assoc Vol 98 Number 5: 357-363, 2008

52. Turek, Samuel L. M.D., Orthopaedics, J. B. Lippincott Co. 1984.

53. Turvey MT, Human movement science 26 (2007) 667-697.

54. Vincent Davis, R., The Tarsal Tunnel Syndrome – A Conservative Approach to Treatment, M.P.I's Dynamic Chiropractic, P. 15, March 26, 1993.

55. Warfel, John H. Ph.D., The Extremities, Lea & Febiger, 1976.

56. Warwick, R., Williams, P., Gray's Anatomy, 35th British Edition, W. B. Saunders Co. 1975.

57. Wyke, Barry, Ph.D., The Neurology of Joints: A Review of General Principles, Clinics in Rheumatic Diseases- Vol. 7, No.1. April 1981, W. B. Saunders Co.

58. Yokum and Rowe. Essentials of Skeletal Radiology, Williams and Wilkins 1988.